INCONTINENCE

Patient Problems and Nursing Care

Marion Moody
MPhil, RGN, RM, Dip Nursing (Lond), RCNT, RNT, BA

Acting Senior Tutor, Professional Development,
Dorset School of Nursing, Poole

Heinemann Nursing

Heinemann Nursing
An imprint of Heinemann Professional Publishing Ltd
Halley Court, Jordan Hill, Oxford OX2 8EJ

OXFORD   LONDON   SINGAPORE   NAIROBI   IBADAN
KINGSTON

First published 1990

British Library Cataloguing in Publication Data
Moody, Marion
    Incontinence.
    1. Incontinent patients. Nursing
    I. Title   II. Series
    610.73'69

ISBN 0 433 00086 4

Photoset by Wilmaset, Birkenhead, Wirral
Printed in Great Britain by Biddles Ltd,
Guildford & Kings Lynn

INCONTINENCE

Patient Problems
and
Nursing Care

Contents

Preface

My primary reason for writing this book is to offer a nursing perspective on incontinence. Several excellent books on this widespread and distressing disorder are already available, but they are incomplete, tending to portray only the medical picture.

Incontinence sufferers spend most of their lives beyond the safety net of the clinic or their counsellor. I have therefore tried first of all to highlight the effects of incontinence on everyday life by illustrating the personal experience of patients, their perceptions of and attitudes towards their situation.

A clear understanding of the relevant normal physiology and pathophysiology of the urinary tracts is essential under-pinning knowledge for effective intervention, and the brief résumé in Chapter 2 leads to an explanation of the physical origins and classification of incontinence. A chapter on patient assessment emphasises the philosophy of self-care as expressed in the writing of Orem (1985). The information obtained from the nursing history and assessment then provides a framework for the nursing intervention. Because the range of treatments and intervention to assist patients regain continence is enormous, guidelines and advice on their most effective use with various client groups are suggested. All chapters have been well referenced and were up to date at the time of writing, but regular scanning of the specialist literature will enlarge and continually refresh this resource.

Teaching strategies and the educative aspect of the nurse's role in the promotion of self-care receive particular attention. Long-term care in the community and meeting the special needs of the elderly, children and disabled with problems of incontinence can prove particular problems. Practical suggestions to resolve these, based on well tried and tested approaches may be useful and open up other avenues for new ideas to emerge.

Two themes that run concurrently through the book relate to a patient centred and multidisciplinary approach in the promotion of continence and the management of incontinence. These are based on the assumption that education about their situation can have a positive influence on an individual's behaviour.

Providing for a better service for patients who are incontinent is one of my long standing interests, both as a practitioner and as an educationalist. As course tutor to the Dorset and Salisbury College of Midwifery and Nursing ENB Course 978, 'The Promotion of Continence and Management of Incontinence', I am able to keep in touch with advances in theoretical and clinical knowledge. In addition, working with a highly motivated and innovative group of people, both colleagues and patients, is intensely rewarding and I continue to learn much from them all. I hope that the experience I have gained will also be of benefit to you and to your patients.

Marion Moody

1

The effects of incontinence on everyday life

INTRODUCTION

All societies have rules – some unwritten – which govern the way people are expected to behave. These rules vary between different societies and usually reflect prevailing cultural norms and values. In our society it is acceptable for a small child to be incontinent of urine and faeces; however, once he or she commences full-time education, incontinence provokes a less acceptable response. Attitudes towards the subject of incontinence and those who suffer from it will be discussed in this chapter.

HUMANS AS RATIONAL BEINGS

Human beings have been described as psychophysical organisms with rational powers; we exist and respond both as organism and object in an environment with physical and biological components. As rationally functioning beings we formulate purposes about the act on ourselves, others, and the environment (Caley et al, 1980). Yet, when faced with the loss of voluntary control of elimination, our actions do not always demonstrate this. For example, when a physical symptom is noticeable and causes fear and alarm to the individual concerned, the normal, rational response is to seek professional help; another way of coping is denial. Incontinence illustrates a good case in point: despite the often obvious signs of incontinence and the devastating effects it can have, many still fail to seek professional help. At times they go to elaborate means to try and conceal the problem. Few nurses working in the community will not have come across this type of situation. It is sometimes extremely difficult to find out why someone wishes to conceal incontinence.

REASONS FOR NOT SEEKING PROFESSIONAL HELP

Fear

Fear is a natural reaction when someone feels he or she is not in control of events happening to them. In some situations fear may incite people to seek help to regain their control or alternatively, it may prompt them to conceal the situation.

For some with incontinence the fear is of not being able to manage independently (Muir-Gray, 1980); that they may be 'put away' or face recrimination if they make a 'mess'. Others may be frightened because they do not know what to expect if they seek help. In elderly people, incontinence may be regarded as a sign of senility, engendering the fear of loss of independence and being taken into care.

Embarrassment

In health, the majority of adults in our society undertake elimination of the body's waste products in the privacy of a toilet. And whilst it is socially acceptable for men to micturate in the presence of each other, women usually perform this function in private. Both sexes are expected to defecate in private.

The loss of control over either or both of these basic functions can and frequently does cause great embarrassment, which may manifest itself in a variety of ways.

Shame

Such is the power of childhood conditioning and cultural expectations that many people feel profoundly ashamed of being incontinent and go to considerable lengths to conceal the problem. It may be that they feel dirty in some way because of soiling themselves or their surroundings.

Denial

Fear, embarrassment, shame or guilt may cause people to deny, even in the face of overwhelming evidence, that they are incontinent. Nurses, especially those working in the community, may be subjected to quite lengthy explanations of odours or wet patches. Soiled garments may be found hidden away in cupboards or drawers, spare rooms or under the stairs.

Resignation

Some people feel a sense of hopelessness and helplessness about their incontinence and resign themselves to the inevitability of the situation, believing in many cases that nothing can be done and that their condition is incurable (Oliver, 1985). These feelings may arise if they feel they are trapped in a physical shell from which no escape seems possible. Unfortunately, some people are actively encouraged to accept their incontinence by health care professionals, even when with correct diagnosis and management continence can be restored. For example, a nurse was overheard to say to a patient who was recovering from a stroke: 'Don't worry about the incontinence, it often happens after a stroke; we'll put a catheter in to keep you dry'. In another situation a lady said she was informed by her general practitioner that she would have to 'learn to live' with her incontinence as nothing could be done due to her age (63 years). Where these attitudes prevail, it is often difficult and time-consuming for a professional carer who has a positive attitude towards incontinence to develop and promote similar attitudes in the patient and negative carers, even when evidence for potential success or more effective management can be demonstrated.

PERSONAL ACCOUNT OF INCONTINENCE

The following case history spans some 11 years and is a personal account by Mrs Jones of how her incontinence problem began and the effect it had on her life. It also highlights the different attitudes of health care professionals towards incontinence and those who suffer from it.

I had my first baby at the age of 34 and the second when I was 37 (in 1966). It was after that pregnancy that I started with bladder problems, which were very minor at first.

On odd occasions I found that for no apparent reason and without warning I wet myself and I could do nothing to stop this. It occurred very infrequently, but I found it a little disconcerting. Whilst I never troubled the doctor unless absolutely necessary, I decided that I should follow the matter up in case, through neglect, I would make matters worse. I visited my doctor and he arranged an appointment for me at the Maternity Clinic. I attended on two occasions, but on examination nothing was found to be amiss and I was told rather brusquely to go home and forget it. In their defence the clinic was extremely busy, but I felt I must have been making a fuss over nothing and I decided it was obviously a small matter and one I would have to live with. I was led to believe it was a common thing to have happened after a pregnancy, especially as I was an older mum.

In 1971 we moved and my recently widowed father was also now living with us, so I was fully occupied, especially as he had arthritis which was slowly getting worse. My initial bladder problem was occurring more frequently and lasting a day or two at a time. I put this down to possible stress caused by my family commitments at the time.

In June 1975, after 5½ years, my father died and I felt that my problem would probably improve with a less demanding life and I would give it time to do so before troubling a doctor again. Despite this change, I found that instead of a gradual improvement there was a decided deterioration and instead of days of inconvenience it was a longer period of a week or 10 days. This could not be stress, surely, especially as I had had a good holiday and rest.

In September 1976 I decided to visit my doctor, choosing the lady doctor in the partnership simply because being a woman she should understand my symptoms more readily. She examined me, said I was 'strong in that area' and could find nothing wrong, so she prescribed some pills to try to resolve the problem. I felt she was sympathetic and she knew from my records that I did not trouble her or her colleagues without good reason.

I kept returning to her at regular intervals for check-ups (always grateful that my appointments did not coincide with an attack). She could not find anything physically wrong and tried different pills. (I realise in retrospect that my muscles were probably strong because I had started to go to keep-fit classes in September 1971, and attended regularly.)

In the meantime, I was having real difficulties during my periods with incontinence. It involved constant personal washing, padding myself up all the time, walking slower when I went out and wearing a mac in case anyone gave me a lift home so I should not wet the car seat. I started to avoid going out if possible and moving quickly. I had a horror of smelling or showing wet patches on my skirts. Any old clothes became the order of the day so as not to spoil better things. Intercourse was often put off because I felt dirty at the time. I told no one – not even my husband – of my plight. As it seemed that there was nothing wrong physically, I began to wonder whether it was something mental and all in the mind at my age. (I was 47 by this time.)

In December 1976, my doctor referred me to a consultant at the local general hospital. He examined me (during a 'good' time). He arranged a visit to x-ray in January 1977. My bladder was filled with a dye and I was x-rayed as it emptied. It was uncomfortable, especially the next day, but was I getting somewhere at last? I was so frustrated, and desperate, and becoming more withdrawn. The result showed some kinks in the bladder and I was admitted for a Marshal Marchetti [a technique for pelvic floor defects] in March 1977. At last, something physical, so it was not a mental problem after all. What a relief – I was beginning to be believed.

Everything went well. I did get an infection after the operation which was very painful but I coped with it. My morale lifted. I was so grateful for the help I was receiving. I was filled with cautious optimism. I promised readily to be careful of what I did when I left hospital 2 weeks later. I did feel rather weak at the time, so I was glad to take as much rest as possible. My husband arranged for temporary domestic help and I limited myself to light work. I did take care. Three months later I stooped to pick something up in the garden and to my consternation a flood of urine shot out on the ground.

At intervals, the old trouble began to start up again. It was as if I had a lidless jar inside me which was spilling over all the time. I talked to my doctor who felt that I had not given myself sufficient time for the muscles to tighten up. She told me to give myself another 3 months to see what happened.

I went on holiday abroad and found myself backing out of accompanying the others, saying I was tired, rather than disclosing the depressing news about myself. I shunned participating in activities as much as I could and I put off going to the doctor because I did not want to be a nuisance and make more fuss. I was driven to doing so by December after weeks and weeks of complete incontinence. She immediately wrote to the consultant – I was reluctant to go, but she said I must. So rather apologetically, because I felt I was casting doubts on his professional skill, I returned to him. He examined me again, said 'cough' and to my utter confusion urine shot out everywhere. He told me everything had collapsed and that he would be able to make a good job for me this time. He told me it must have been rotten for me and he would get me admitted as soon as possible after Christmas. He was very understanding and encouraging, which helped my confidence a great deal. True to his word I was admitted 3 weeks later, 10 months after the first operation. I was cured – after 12 years.

Even though it is now 9 years since this time, I still feel the tremendous gratitude I felt at that time and I do not think I shall ever take my controlled bladder for granted again.

Incontinence made me very self-conscious and withdrawn. I just wanted to crawl away. I missed playing rushing about games with my children. I became isolated and lonely in my struggle and it caused me much mental anguish and heart-searching.

Having read Mrs Jones's personal account of life during her period of incontinence, do you think anything could have been done earlier to help her?

Unfortunately, there are many thousands of people who, like Mrs Jones, experience the mental anguish of incontinence. Research findings (Thomas et al, 1980) have suggested that a high proportion of these people never seek the professional help they so desperately require. It must therefore be the responsibility of the professionals to create an atmosphere which encourages people to seek help.

In the majority of circumstances incontinence can be cured with appropriate treatment. It is only a minority of people who remain incontinent despite treatment, and even in these cases effective management can enhance the quality of their lives and those of their carers and families.

Many people who are incontinent find themselves severely limited in the activities that form part of the general pattern of life. In some instances what should be an enjoyable experience becomes filled with anxiety and frustration which, if not sensitively handled, could lead to depression and despair.

ACTIVITIES WHICH MAY BE AFFECTED BY INCONTINENCE

1 Making journeys.
2 Shopping.
3 Playing games or sports.
4 Dancing.
5 Attending school or work.
6 Going on holiday.
7 Forming relationships.
8 Socializing.
9 Wearing certain types of clothing.
10 Family life.

Journeys

For those who are continent, journeys pose few problems. For a person who is incontinent the thought of venturing outside the door may cause such panic and fear that the journey is ended before it begins. For those who do venture out, the journey may be full of hazards unless it is well planned. What route, for example, must be taken if regular toilet facilities are required? What contingency plans must be made if one or more of the public lavatories is out of action? How can accidents be avoided? Is there going to be a problem over the disposal of soiled pads or pants? Can the problem be overcome? Will assistance be required and will it be available? Will there be sufficient room for another person in the lavatory, should assistance be required? Sometimes it is impossible to find a suitable toilet for a wheelchair (Baroness Marsham of Ilton, 1985). For many people, journeys are restricted to within the locality of known toilet facilities.

Shopping

Public lavatories are not always evident in many shopping areas, and there are many shops which do not provide facilities for shoppers to use on the premises. Hence shopping expeditions may require careful planning, especially when people have urge incontinence or frequency of micturition. Those with stress incontinence may find they have to be aware of the weight of their shopping bags, and take extra care when bending to lift boxes or bags from trolleys or cars and when carrying goods into the home.

Some people worry when in close proximity to others in case any unpleasant odours or damp patches are noticed, especially whilst they are waiting in queues.

Sport

Activity, even mild activity, can precipitate an uncontrolled episode of leakage. Such accidents as a rule are not well tolerated by those who witness the events. This is primarily due to our deeply ingrained cultural taboos on elimination. The person who has suffered this type of experience is often deeply upset and feels so ashamed that such activities are not engaged in again.

Dancing

Dancing is also an activity which can precipitate incontinence and therefore some people who become incontinent give up their dancing for fear of having an accident. Withdrawal from normal recreational activities can lead many incontinent people to feelings of social isolation and despair.

Attending school or work

The lives of many adults and children are often made quite intolerable because of incontinence. Children who wet or soil themselves at school are frequently subject to ridicule by their peers and chastised by their teachers and even parents. Such attitudes can have a profound psychological and emotional effect, which may remain with them throughout their lives and can result in the development of behavioural problems.

Unfortunately, even when a child is known to have a physical or mental disability which results in a lack of control over excretory functions, those around are not always understanding or tolerant of the situation.

Work can also cause its share of misery for someone who has incontinence or suffers from frequency of micturition. For some people, the termination of their employment becomes a reality. Consider the situation of David, a young man of 29 who suffered from frequency of micturition. After being warned by his employer about the number of visits he made to the washroom during the day he was dismissed. The results of his employer's action caused him great financial and psychological embarrassment.

Others may be faced with the constant threat of discovery through unpleasant odours or telltale stains and damp patches. Disposal of soiled garments or concealment of replacement ones can be a problem for some people, especially if space for storing personal items is very restricted.

The range and type of work may have to be limited if leakage is to be avoided or if frequent interruption of the job is not possible or permissible. Even those with an obvious disability, such as paraplegia, may not always find it easy to manage their appliance at work or ask for help (Borthwick, 1985).

Holidays

Holidays are something that most people look forward to with great delight. However, for many incontinent people the thought of going on holiday is never even contemplated because it generates so much anxiety and fear because of the risk of having their incontinence discovered through accidents occurring in public places.

Of those who feel able to venture on holiday, many still experience anxiety over the risk of wet beds, spillage on the floor, damp patches on furniture and methods for disposing of soiled garments or used appliances. One problem that frequently arises is related to pads. People who use pads when going away on holiday find these items very bulky to transport. Whilst it is now possible to purchase additional supplies of pads and pants from many chemists across the country, the cost incurred can be very high for the individuals concerned. As yet no arrangements exist where free supplies can be obtained from a different health authority for the duration of a holiday.

This type of problem may be overcome by changing the method of incontinence management, but only if the patient consents. However, experience often shows that even when patients and their families are willing to try an alternative form of management, this may not be supported by health care professionals.

For example, intermittent self-catheterization may be the preferred method of management of both patient and family. Margaret is a typical example of someone who met with strong opposition from professional carers over her desire to be taught to use intermittent self-catheterization in preparation for her holiday.

Margaret was 32 when she was involved in an accident which left her paraplegic. Previously she had led an active life and worked as a private secretary. After being discharged from the spinal injuries unit, both Margaret and her husband decided that they would have as near normal private and social life as possible within the constraints of Margaret's disability. This they did successfully with one exception. Both wanted to recommence taking their holidays abroad and all problems over accommodation and transport arrangements had been resolved. However, Margaret felt that the quantity of pads and pants required for a 10-day holiday would be too bulky to transport. She therefore approached her general practitioner and community nurse with a view to being taught how to catheterize herself. Her husband was also prepared to learn the technique should Margaret ever be unable to carry out the necessary procedure. Unfortunately, neither the doctor nor the community nurse were in favour of this technique and offered in its place a temporary indwelling catheter or the continuation of her present pads and pants. The alternative was not acceptable to either Margaret or her husband and both were left feeling angry and frustrated that their attempts at normalcy were being thwarted by professional 'carers'.

The controversy surrounding intermittent catheterization is discussed in detail in Chapter 5. The importance of the involvement of patients and relatives in deciding on appropriate management must be stressed; the final decision on any treatment or management should be the patient's, whenever possible.

Relationships and socialization

Socialization is an interactive process by which individuals adopt the prevailing attitudes, values and cultural practices of their group. If this process is satisfactory then the individual is usually able to function as an acceptable member of that group in the roles he or she adopts throughout life. It may be that those who are incontinent have been socialized into believing they are deviant and therefore different from those who retain their continence. Such attitudes often make it difficult for those with incontinence to form and develop meaningful relationships, and can result in feelings of desolation and despair.

Some incontinent people see life as a vicious circle, fearing rejection for concealing or highlighting their problems. Neil was 19 and still had episodes of nocturnal enuresis. His mother only contacted their general practitioner when she realized that her son wanted to get engaged. When Neil came for his appointment it became apparent that he was extremely anxious about the thought of telling his girlfriend of his problem in case she not only rejected him, but also told their friends. Happily this situation had a satisfactory ending.

Unfortunately there are numerous situations where what little self-confidence and esteem individuals have left is undermined, driving them even more into solitude.

Clothing

There are many people like Mrs Jones who resort to wearing old clothes, rather than risk soiling their better ones. The constant wearing of old clothes can however result in a lowering of self-esteem and pride in appearance. Some people with incontinence feel afraid to wear shorts or swimwear, or lightweight flimsy garments in case any appliance or incontinence pad shows through, or soiled undergarments become visible. Fabrics vary considerably in quality and some materials and colours tend to show up any damp patches more than others. As a basic rule, black appears to be a good colour to wear as it tends to disguise damp patches.

Family life

Incontinence has already been shown to affect all members of a family. Mrs Jones mentioned not only her inability to play many of the children's games with them, but also the sexual side of her marriage. The fear that urine or faeces might leak during a sexual act can severely inhibit the incontinent partner, and may lead them to decline any form of sexual advancement. This may ultimately leave the other partner feeling frustrated, angry and confused at being rejected.

Even when both partners know of the risk of leakage, problems can still arise. Firstly, the thought of leakage could result in the continent partner feeling repelled at the prospect, reducing sexual libido. Secondly, both partners may become anxious about any potential mishap, introducing tension into their relationship.

Family life can also be disrupted if there is a reluctance by the incontinent member to attend social functions. Alternatively, the reluctance could be on the part of the family either to include the incontinent relative or to allow entertainment in the home for fear of embarrassing accidents.

Children who fail to attain continence by the expected age can also be a source of stress within the family (Turner, 1987).

An even greater strain can be placed upon the family when, for example, an elderly relative's behaviour has become unbearable. (Swaffield, 1981). Impairment of mental function with age may lead to a person eliminating on the floor or in inappropriate receptacles like hand basins or bowls. Some people with severe mental function impairment (such as advanced dementia) have a tendency to smear excreta around their environment. Such behaviour causes great distress to the family, which is quite understandable and necessitates the patient receiving expert medical assessment, whilst the relatives need support and guidance from the primary health care team. A few individuals are also obsessed with wrapping up excreta or soiled garments into small parcels and hiding them in a variety of sites, mainly cupboards, drawers, wardrobes and the like, which again can be very distressing for the person finding the item.

THE FINANCIAL IMPLICATIONS OF INCONTINENCE

Incontinence can cause severe financial hardship to individuals and their families, especially when they have not sought professional advice. Many people who are incontinent resort to using sanitary pads which, apart from the expense, are totally unsuitable for containing leakage.

Unfortunately this situation is often made worse by a lack of knowledge on the part of professionals as to the appropriate aid to contain the problem whilst a treatment programme is being planned. Some people, although known to be incontinent, are still expected in certain health districts to contribute a considerable amount of money towards their management, and not all management aids are available on an FP10 form.

ATTITUDES OF THOSE WITH INCONTINENCE TOWARDS THEIR SITUATION

It is essential that health care professionals and significant others in a person's life have an accurate understanding of that person's attitudes towards the incontinence. It is only then that factors which may help or hinder continence promotion or the effective management of incontinence can be clearly identified and acted upon.

The following is a summary of attitudes of individuals towards their incontinence:

1 Fear.
2 Embarrassment.

3 Shame.
4 Guilt.
5 Hostility.
6 Resentment.
7 Anger.
8 Frustration.
9 Hopelessness.
10 Helplessness.
11 Acceptance.
12 Apathy.
13 Revulsion.
14 Denial.

ATTITUDES OF HEALTH CARE PROFESSIONALS AND SIGNIFICANT OTHERS

Incontinence can provoke a range of attitudes in both health care professionals and significant others which may create major obstacles in promoting continence or managing incontinence more effectively. In principle, most nurses feel they should be able to cope with their patient's symptoms and nursing demands. It can, therefore, be very difficult for nurses to feel able to express attitudes like revulsion, anger, and frustration when faced with incontinence. Alternatively, nurses may adopt attitudes towards their patient which appear condescending or patronizing, telling patients, for example, not to worry about being incontinent as it happens a lot, or saying things like: 'There is plenty of linen or clean clothes available'.

Despite changes within the profession, largely brought about through education, there still remains a large proportion of nurses who believe nothing can be done about incontinence; that it is an inevitable part of growing old or being handicapped. Another problem in improving this situation is a lack of awareness of the number of people who may be incontinent. A postal survey covering a number of different locations was conducted by Thomas et al (1980); more than 18 000 responses were received. The definition for incontinence was given as 'involuntary leakage of urine in inappropriate places or at inappropriate times twice or more a month' – regardless of the quantity of urine lost! The findings indicated that between two and three million people within the UK may suffer from regular incontinence (Table 1.1).

Table 1.1. Prevalence of regular urinary incontinence

| Sex | [Age (years)] | |
	15–64	65+
Male	1.6%	6.9%
Female	8.5%	11.6%

From Thomas et al (1980).

It is evident from the findings of Thomas et al (1980) that incontinence in females is higher both in the 15–64 and the over 65 age group. Approximately 1 in 4 women and 1 in 10 men appear to suffer from regular incontinence. Disturbing as this may be, the study revealed that of the total population who indicated they were incontinent, only a tiny proportion were known to be incontinent by the health, social or voluntary bodies and were receiving any form of help (Table 1.2).

Table 1.2. Prevalence of urinary incontinence known to health, social and voluntary bodies

| Sex | [Age (years)] | |
	15–64	65+
Male	0.1%	1.3%
Female	0.2%	2.5%

From Thomas et al (1980).

For those wishing to know more about prevalence studies and attitudes towards incontinence, further reading is given at the end of this chapter.

In order to improve the current situation nurses need to have a much greater understanding of the prevalence of incontinence and be encouraged to discuss their own feelings, attitudes and bias on incontinence with their peers in a structured and meaningful manner. Then they will be more able to help patients, relatives and other carers to identify and discuss their attitudes towards what is described as one of the most distressing and disabling symptoms known to afflict western society.

References

Baroness Marsham of Ilton (1985). Keeping to a routine. *Nursing Times*, April 3, 85 (14), 71.
Borthwick J. (1985). Speaking from experience. *Nursing Times*, April 3, 85 (14), 69.
Caley J. M., Dirkman M., Engalla M. et al (1980). The Orem self care nursing model. In *Conceptual Models for Nursing*. (Riehl J. P., Callister R., eds). London: Appleton Century and Croft.
Muir-Gray J. A. (1980). Incontinence in the community. In *Incontinence and its Management*. (Mandelstam D., ed.). London: Croom Helm.
Oliver J. (1985). Fresh and dry. *Nursing Times*, July 24, 81 (30), 4.
Swaffield L. (1981). Attitudes to incontinence. *Nursing Times*, February 12, 77 (7), 51–61.
Turner A. F. (1987). Childhood continence problems. *Professional Nurse*, 2 (4), 119–21.
Thomas T. M., Playmat K. R., Blannin J. et al (1980). The prevalence of urinary incontinence. *British Medical Journal*, 281, 1243–5.

Bibliography

Bradshaw J. (1978). *Incontinence – A Burden for Families with Handicapped Children*. London: Disabled Living Foundation.
Hamilton B. (1988). Education for continence. *Nursing Times*, 84 (14), 78, 82.
Harris J. (1984). Positive step. *Nursing Mirror*, February 15, 158 (7).
Rooney V. (1985). How would you manage? *Nursing Times*, April 3, 81 (14), 65–6.
Rowell T. J. (1980). *Problems in Geriatric Nursing Care*. Edinburgh: Churchill Livingstone.

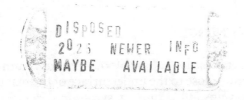
2

The bladder: physiology and pathophysiology

The bladder has one main function – to act as a reservoir for urine. Anatomically it is frequently described as a hollow pear-shaped organ situated in the pelvic cavity which gradually becomes ovoid in shape when filling with urine. It's four surfaces lie in close proximity to other organs of the body:

1 The anterior surface is separated from the symphysis pubis by a pad of fat.
2 On the superior surface there are coils of small intestine.
3 The posterior (commonly referred to as the base of the bladder) and the inferior surface relate to different organs in the male and female. In the male the posterior surface of the bladder lies close to the rectum and seminal vesicles, whereas in the female it is adjacent to the uterus. The prostate gland and urethra adjoin the inferior surface in the male and in the female the urethra fascia and muscles of the pelvic floor adjoin the inferior surface.
4 A layer of peritoneum partially covers the superior bladder surface.

BLOOD SUPPLY

The bladder receives its blood supply from the vesical branches of the internal iliac arteries. In the female the vaginal and uterine arteries also supply blood. Venous return is via the plexus of vessels close to the undersurface of the bladder to the internal iliac veins.

NERVE SUPPLY

Current theories of bladder innervation and control remain contradictory (Brocklehurst, 1984). The following account is therefore a simplification; the nerve supply is further discussed in Chapter 3. Readers who wish to know more about bladder innervation are directed to the literature detailed at the end of this chapter.

Autonomic and somatic nerves supply both the bladder and urethra. The autonomic supply is via the hypogastric plexus situated at the linea terminalis of the pelvis and consists of sympathetic and parasympathetic nerves. The sympathetic outflow has its origins in the grey matter of the first, second and probably third lumbar segments of the spinal cord where special neurone cells are found. The nerve fibres travel through the coeliac and mesenteric ganglia to form the presacral nerve which lies in front of the bladder (Fig. 2.1). The sympathetic nerves then innervate the bladder base and sphincters at the bladder neck.

The parasympathetic nerves are the key motor nerves to the detrusor muscle and bladder neck sphincters. They arise from the second and third sacral cord segments, as shown in Fig. 2.1. Nerve impulses are transmitted along the white preganglionic fibres via the nervi erigentes to the hypogastric ganglia, where they synapse and travel along the grey postganglionic fibres to the bladder. Here they synapse with neurone cells in the bladder.

The conduction of nerve impulses is facilitated by the liberation of a chemical substance called acetylcholine at the pre- and post-ganglionic junction. Acetylcholine is also released at the parasympathetic nerve endings, whereas noradrenaline is released at the sympathetic nerve endings. (Figs 2.2 and 2.3).

The main function of the sympathetic nerves is to close the sphincters round the bladder neck and relax the bladder. The

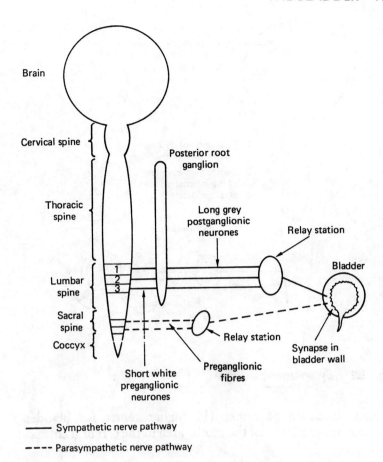

Fig. 2.1. *Sympathetic and parasympathetic nerve pathway.*

parasympathetic nerve stimulates contraction of the bladder muscle and relaxation of the sphincters. The somatic nerves also originate from the second and third sacral segments of the spinal cord. They supply the striated (voluntary) muscles of the pelvic floor. The most important of the nerves are the pudendal. Sensory information from the bladder, urethra and pelvic floor is relayed via these somatic nerves.

The pudendal nerves facilitate contraction of the pelvic floor and voluntary closure of the external urethra sphincter if urine flow is to be interrupted, for example, to obtain a mid-

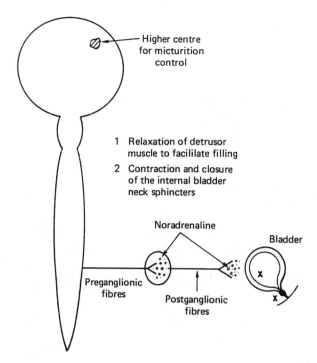

Fig. 2.2. Sympathetic outflow.

stream specimen of urine. The higher centre for bladder control lies at the top of the motor area in the cerebral cortex.

BLADDER STRUCTURE

The walls of the bladder comprise four different tissue types:

1 An outer layer of parietal peritoneum which is incomplete, lying only on the superior and posterior surface.
2 A muscle layer, which consists of three interlacing sets of smooth muscle fibres, collectively called the detrusor muscle. The contractile properties of the muscles accommodates the changing shape of the bladder during filling or voiding. The detrusor is primarily a parasympathetic organ, therefore the major portion of its innervation is

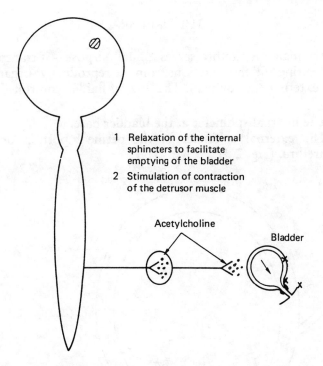

1 Relaxation of the internal
  sphincters to facilitate
  emptying of the bladder
2 Stimulation of contraction
  of the detrusor muscle

Acetylcholine

Bladder

Fig. 2.3. *Parasympathetic outflow.*

cholinergic, although some sympathetic receptors can be found at the apex of the bladder.

3 A submucous layer made up of blood and lymph vessels, sympathetic and parasympathetic nerves, supported in a network of areolar tissue.

4 An inner layer of transitional epithelium forms a mucous membrane, which in health appears a pinkish rose colour. This inner layer of tissue is arranged to form folds called rugae, apparent when the bladder contains only a small volume of urine.

There are three orifices in the bladder wall. Two are formed by the entry of the ureters at an oblique angle of the posterior surface, the third by the exit of the urethra at the bladder neck on the inferior surface. These three orifices form a triangle called the trigone.

THE URETHRA

In the male the urethra serves a dual purpose – it transports both urine and the secretions from the reproductive organs to the external environment. The flow of fluid is controlled by:

1 The internal sphincter at the bladder base.
2 The external sphincter at the perineal portion of the urethra. (Fig. 2.4).

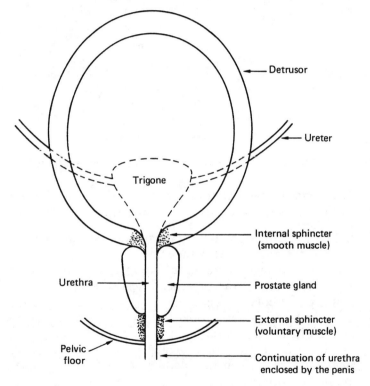

Detrusor

Ureter

Trigone

Internal sphincter
(smooth muscle)

Urethra

Prostate gland

External sphincter
(voluntary muscle)

Pelvic floor

Continuation of urethra
enclosed by the penis

Fig. 2.4. *The internal and external sphincters in the male.*

In the female, the internal sphincter is located at the opening at the bladder neck. The external sphincter is in the perineal section of the urethra (Fig. 2.5). Adequate com-

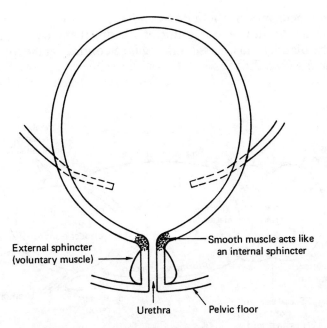

External sphincter
(voluntary muscle)

Smooth muscle acts like
an internal sphincter

Urethra   Pelvic floor

Fig. 2.5.   *The internal and external sphincters in the female.*

pression of the mucosal folds of the urethra provides the watertight closure necessary for maintaining continence (Feneley, 1980).

PHYSIOLOGY OF MICTURITION

One of the things that humans have in common with other animals is our inability to control excretion of urine and faeces at birth. The skill required to attain continence is developed under 'normal' conditions within 3 to 4 years of birth.

Initially micturition results from a reflex action. Urine collecting in the bladder stimulates the stretch and pain receptor cells contained within its walls; this causes sensory nerve impulses to be transmitted to a specialized area (sacral bladder centre) in the posterior root of the second, third and fourth sacral segments. Here they synapse with a special connector cell. The nerve impulses are then transmitted via the motor neurones in the anterior horn cells along the motor pathways to the urethral sphincter, causing them to relax, and to the bladder muscle, stimulating it to contract and expel its contents (Fig. 2.6).

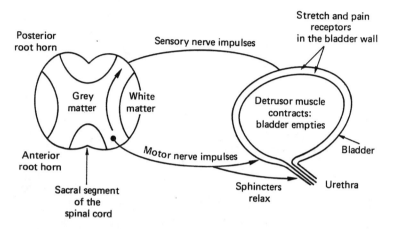

Fig. 2.6. *Sacrospinal reflex arc.*

During maturation the infant becomes increasingly aware of the body and its functions. The higher centre for bladder control in the cerebral cortex becomes involved in the process of micturition and the child gradually learns to inhibit the sacral reflex arc, and hence micturition, until a convenient time and place are found (Fig. 2.7).

This voluntary control is highly complex and requires the infant firstly to be able to recognize that the sensory impulses from the bladder to the brain indicate a full bladder. Secondly, it requires the infant to exercise control and block the reflex arc voluntarily (as described above) by inhibiting motor activity until an appropriate time. Thirdly, the child must consciously remove the inhibition so that micturition may occur. Eventually these conscious processes become automatic under 'normal' conditions.

The bladder, like many other organs of the body, has a complex feedback system to enhance its efficiency (Fig. 2.8).

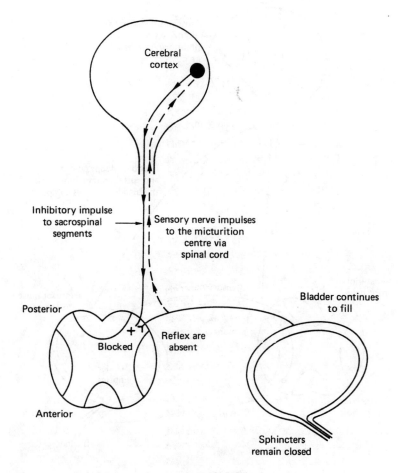

Fig. 2.7.   *Inhibition of sacrospinal reflex arc.*

The mechanism between the bladder and brain is designed to ensure that the sphincters remain open and relaxed and the bladder sustains contraction until it is empty.

NORMAL PATTERNS OF MICTURITION

Patterns of micturition in adults are extremely varied yet may still be classified as normal. They may be influenced by social, cultural, or occupational factors. For example, lectures, bus

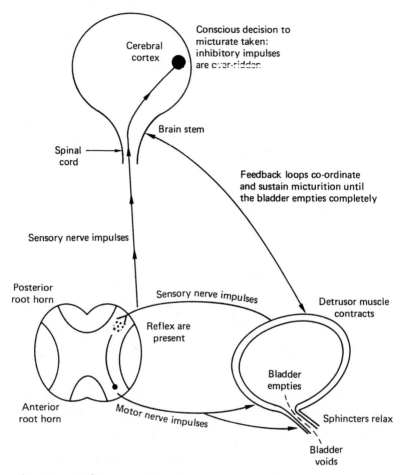

Fig. 2.8. *Voluntary micturition.*

journeys, work or play activities would be constantly inter-rupted if individuals could not exercise voluntary control over their desire to micturate.

BLADDER CAPACITY

The 'average' bladder holds approximately 350–600 ml but it is a well established fact that many people void urine before and after these amounts have been reached with no apparent physical or psychological trauma.

As the bladder fills there is stimulation of the bladder pressure receptors which transmit impulses to the sacral bladder centre in the spinal cord and eventually to the bladder centre in the cerebral cortex of the brain, giving rise to the conscious desire to micturate. When it is inconvenient, the inhibition centre in the cerebral cortex takes over, causing the desire to diminish and the bladder muscle to distend as the intravesical pressure is lowered until a convenient time arises. Alternatively, voluntary emptying of the bladder can arise without the desire to micturate being present.

ACCESSORY ORGANS OF MICTURITION

Increased intra-abdominal pressure is of great assistance to micturition as it leads to compression of the bladder. This is achieved by contraction of the chest wall, resulting in the descent of the diaphragm. In addition closure of the glottis and breath-holding help increase intra-abdominal pressure.

DYSFUNCTION OF MICTURITION

Micturition is a function which is rarely considered by the continent person; it only becomes significant when the mechanism for maintaining continence fails or dysfunctions in some way.

Variation from normal patterns of micturition may result in the symptom which we term incontinence. Incontinence can be defined as the voiding of urine at an inappropriate time and place.

There is a percentage of the population who, for a variety of reasons, have never acquired the skills necessary to control micturition. Others may experience a breakdown of their control mechanisms but, whatever the cause, the results are often devastating to individuals and their families.

CLASSIFICATION OF INCONTINENCE

Writers have classified incontinence in various ways. For the purpose of this book the causes of incontinence will be discussed under two main categories – predisposing factors which have physical origin and precipitating factors such as environmental, social and psychological conditions.

Physical origins of incontinence

The bladder acts primarily as a reservoir for urine until its contents can be voided in an appropriate place. A high proportion of people who suffer from incontinence have some degree of bladder dysfunction. Again classification is arbitrary.

Atonic bladder

This occurs when there has been damage to the sensory nerve pathway between the bladder and sacral segments of the spinal cord. This results in the absence of, or diminished conscious sensation of, bladder fullness, loss of the reflex arc and consequently, reflex micturition.

Consider for a moment the practical implications of this situation (see Table 2.1). Although it may still be possible to micturate voluntarily, the bladder would probably require manual expression and abdominal muscle involvement to empty. This results in the bladder becoming over-distended with volumes of 500–2 000 ml being present and causing, in many instances, overflow incontinence. Frequency of micturition may also be a feature when some degree of sensation is present.

An atonic bladder may develop as a result of a person having tabes dorsalis (very rare today in the UK), sacrospinal metastases, diabetic neuropathy or any other condition which destroys the sacral nerve cells and surrounding tissues.

Bladder instability

Bladder instability may also be referred to as detrusor instability or uninhibited bladder. With this disorder there is a loss of the normal cortical inhibition impulses to the bladder, although the sensation of fullness may be present.

Once again, consider the practical implications (see Fig. 2.6). In the absence of inhibiting impulses from the brain the

Table 2.1. Main causes and types of incontinence

Cerebral
Inflammatory changes
Disseminated sclerosis
Parkinson's disease
Arterial degeneration
Trauma
Mental deficiency
Cerebral tumours
Cerebral vascular accident

Spinal cord
Meningomyelocele
Sacral tumour
Inflammatory disease
Spinal cord compression
Trauma
Demyelinating diseases

Peripheral nerve impairment
Pelvic tumour
Pelvic trauma
Subacute combined degeneration of the spinal cord
Infection
Meningomyelocele
Peripheral neuropathy – diabetes
Disseminated sclerosis

Genitourinary tract
Congenital lesions
Infection
Urethral obstruction
Incompetent sphincter neck
Unstable detrusor muscle
Underactive detrusor muscle
Urethral stricture
Trauma

Miscellaneous
Weak pelvic floor muscles
Impaired mobility or dexterity
Drugs, especially anticholinergic drugs
Psychological factors
Constipation
Environmental factors

sacral reflex arc is often completed before the person can reach the toilet. This situation results in a poor bladder capacity of less than 200 ml. Accompanied by frequency and urgency, the amounts of urine passed are often quite small. The awareness of the desire to micturate, coupled with the inability to 'hold on' until a toilet is reached, often, understandably, causes intense emotional upset to the person concerned.

Research findings, particularly from work by Brocklehurst (1984), have suggested that advancing age is associated with altered patterns of micturition and that most elderly people suffer from some degree of bladder instability. One of the causes may be an upper motor neurone lesion such as a cerebrovascular accident. There is some evidence that young boys are more prone to suffer from unstable bladders than girls, whereas the reverse would appear to be the case in young adults. In some cases there is no apparent neurological dysfunction to explain detrusor instability (Stanton, 1984) and the term idiopathic instability is used to distinguish sufferers from those who can be provided with a reason for their condition.

Stress incontinence

The International Continence Society (1976) has defined stress incontinence as 'the involuntary loss of urine from the urethra when the intravesical pressure exceeds the maximum urethral pressure but in the absence of detrusor activity'. In other words, the urethral sphincter is incompetent and allows urine to leak, especially during periods of physical exertion.

Stress incontinence can occur in males and females, although it is more common in women, due to their short urethra. Some girls are born with a congenital weakness of the sphincter mechanism; others suffer traumatic injury to the bladder neck and surrounding tissues during childbirth, especially when there has been a prolonged second stage or mechanical delivery.

During embryonic life the trigone and urethra are derived from the same tissues as the vagina. After the menopause some women have a tendency to develop senile vaginitis as a result of hormonal deficiency. The atrophic changes which occur also effect the urethra and trigone. This, coupled with relaxation of the pelvic muscles, can lead to frequency and incontinence.

Stress incontinence in men may result from trauma to the urethra sphincter from surgery or other injury.

Outflow obstruction

Outflow obstruction is likely to involve the bladder neck. Whenever an obstruction arises in a muscular organ, the body's natural response is initially to try to overcome the obstruction by increasing the force of its contractions. The detrusor muscle of the bladder may act in this manner producing extremely powerful contractions in its attempt to overcome the outflow obstruction. In many instances the attempt fails, the bladder becomes increasingly distended, the detrusor hypertrophies and exceeds its limits of compliance, causing an atonic bladder to develop. If this situation is not corrected it may lead to impairment of the upper urinary tract and renal function; alternatively, it may give rise to detrusor instability.

Outflow obstruction is typified by the middle-aged or elderly man with chronic retention, who starts wetting the bed at night or finds that he is wet without any sensation of the need to void (Feneley, 1980).

Other symptoms may include:

1 Difficulty in commencing outflow.
2 Dribbling after micturition.
3 Dysuria.
4 Frequency.
5 Hesitancy.
6 Infection.
7 Involuntary leakage of urine.
8 Poor urine flow.
9 Straining.
10 Urgency and urge incontinence.

Outflow obstruction may be caused by a variety of conditions in either sex; the most common cause in men is hypertrophy of the prostate gland. In women outflow obstruction may be due to obstetric complications. Other causes include:

1 Congenital abnormalities.
2 Catheterization or other instrumentation of the urethra.
3 Detrusor sphincter dyssynergia, due to a neurological abnormality usually associated with a traumatic lesion to the upper spinal cord, which causes a simultaneous uncoordinated contraction of the detrusor and urethra, resulting in obstruction to urine outflow. Under normal conditions the urethra relaxes as the detrusor contracts.
4 Tumours involving the bladder neck, post-surgical complications following hypospadias repair or prostatectomy.
5 Urethritis.
6 Sexually transmitted disease.

Precipitating factors
Infection of the urinary tract

Infection can be a precipitating factor in causing incontinence either on its own or in association with other conditions. Infection is more common in females than males due to women's short urethras. Brocklehurst and Dillane (1967) suggested that the age-related changes which occur in the lower urinary tract and pelvis reduce resistance to infection. A proportion of elderly people who have a chronic urinary infection also have incontinence. The presence of residual urine increases the risk of infection, as does the introduction of a urethral catheter.

Infection of the urinary tract may present in many different ways. The patient may be asymptomatic or have atypical symptoms such as abdominal or loin pains and painless haematuria without alteration of micturating pattern. More commonly the presenting symptoms include urgency and urge incontinence, frequency, dysuria, unpleasant odour of urine, subrapubic and/or loin pain and pyrexia. *Escherichia coli* is the most commonly found organism invading the urinary tract, followed by *Proteus mirabilis* and other types of non *E. coli* coliforms.

Psuedomonas, *Streptococcus faecalis* and *Klebsiella* are often isolated following instrumentation or catheterization of the urinary tract. It is vital to pay particular attention to asepsis during these and other such procedures.

Faecal impaction and urinary incontinence

Faecal impaction occurs as a result of chronic constipation. Normally faecal matter is propelled along the colon by peristalsis towards the anal canal for evacuation. During its journey through the transverse and descending colon, fluid is absorbed thus reducing the size of the mass. Defecation normally occurs when voluntary and involuntary action are jointly initiated by the passage of faeces into the rectum. The conscious desire to defecate can be inhibited by contraction of the external anal sphincters if it is not convenient to proceed; however, frequent inhibiting of the natural defecation reflexes or damage to the nerve pathways can result in constipation.

There are two types of impaction – pultaceous and scybalous. Pultaceous is less common and consists of large quantities of putty-like faecal matter in the distal colon. Scybalous is more common and consists of hard faecal masses (scybala) in the rectum, which have a tendency to irritate the mucosa of the colon causing it to produce copious amounts of mucus. This, together with the faecal fluid from the proximal part of the colon, can leak past the scybala producing spurious diarrhoea and faecal incontinence.

It is important to consider whether faecal impaction will affect bladder function. The effects vary according to the severity of the condition, for example, constant straining at constipated stools can lead to over-stretching and weakness of the pelvic floor muscles, thereby predisposing the person to stress incontinence. Distension in the pelvic region could also interfere with normal nerve conduction as well as causing direct pressure on the bladder and urethra, resulting in outflow obstruction. The affects of general malaise and lethargy must not be underestimated and will be discussed later in the book.

Drugs

There are several categories of drugs which affect bladder function. The obvious example is the diuretics which substantially increase urinary output. In some instances the patient may be unable to 'hold on' until reaching the toilet, the result being urge incontinence. The patient's difficulties may be compounded by restrictions in mobility due to, for example, arthritis (Judd, 1989). Other categories of drugs include those used in the treatment of respiratory, cardiac, gastric, neurological and psychological disorders; anti-depressants and anti-hypertensives can affect the smooth muscle of the bladder and sphincters. Thus we may summarize the main side-effects of drugs on bladder function as causing voiding problems and the risk of retention of urine. The exceptions are drugs such as methyldopa which can act upon the smooth muscle of the detrusor and urethra to cause stress incontinence. Some of these drugs can also have a therapeutic effect, for example, propranolol and salbutamol can both help alleviate stress incontinence.

Psychological factors

Various studies of incontinence have revealed the presence of a number of different emotional or mental states which appear to contribute to its development (Menninger, 1941; Schwartz and Stanton, 1950; Palmtag and Reidasch 1980; Yarnell et al, 1982).

Menninger (1941) identified the presence of neuroticism in some children and elderly people who had polyuria. Yarnell et al (1982) found that women who had urge and a combination of urge and stress incontinence scored higher than average on the neuroticism scale. It is not, however, clear if neuroticism precipitates incontinence, or if the incontinence precipitates neurosis. Palmtag and Reidasch (1980) concluded from their urodynamic studies on 1300 patients that 2.7% had alterations of voiding patterns due to psychosis or neurosis.

Others have postulated that incontinence is a feature of anxiety or emotional breakdown and may follow a sudden life crisis such as a traumatic illness or bereavement. The association between anxiety and urgency is well known. The queues of people waiting to use the toilet on examination days is a common feature in schools – and colleges of nursing! The act of incontinence has given rise to some people being labelled as attention-seeking, troublesome and retaliative, disruptive, manipulative or depressive. There are considerable qualitative data to suggest that incontinence does have a depressive effect on many sufferers. The need for carers and professionals to adopt a positive but realistic approach to the situation cannot be over-stated.

Where there is considered to be impairment of mental function due to disease or trauma, associated with incontinence, there often exists a high level of acceptance that nothing can be done about improving the situation, distasteful though it may be to the carers and in many instances, to the incontinent person as well. In practice much can be done to help many people regain continence, and where this is not feasible, considerable help can be offered to improve incontinence management.

Newly hospitalized elderly people may become incontinent simply as a result of confusion and disorientation. Reality orientation is essential to combat the confusing effects of admission and help prevent incontinence.

Explanation, reassurance, and careful assessment of the patient's drug regime can do much to alleviate or minimize confusion. Attention should also be paid to the patients' social environment, to ensure that they do not feel socially isolated or demotivated. A loss of self-esteem will make continence a much more difficult goal for the patient to achieve.

Geographical factors

The geographical surroundings within which a person may live – be it their own home, a nursing home or a hospital – may not be conducive to maintaining or regaining continence. In many instances the toilets are not easily accessible or readily available and if the person also suffers from problems of mobility it may make the negotiation of stairs or moving any distance an additional handicap which can result in incontinence. The lack of privacy when wishing to use the toilet or comode, especially in communal accommodation, may also precipitate bladder or bowel dysfunction.

The situation is further aggravated at night when the lights are dim and patients cannot easily attract the attention of a nurse without making a noise or ringing a bell, which they may be reluctant to do for fear of disturbing other patients.

For some people the physical and psychological effort

required to maintain continence is great. Without motivation, self-esteem and encouragement, patients may give in to what they consider to be their inevitable fate – the development of incontinence. However, in all of the situations referred to in this section it is possible to improve the quality of life for the patient. Exactly how this can be done is discussed later in the book.

References

Brocklehurst J. C. (1984). *Urology in the Elderly.* Edinburgh: Churchill Livingstone.
Brocklehurst J. C., Dillane J. B. (1967). Studies of the female bladder in old age: micturating cystograms in incontinent women. *Gerontologia Clinica*, 9, 47–58.
Feneley R. C. L. (1980). Normal micturition and its control. In *Incontinence and its Management* (Mandelstam D., ed.) London: Croom Helm.
Feneley R. C. L. (1980). Urological aspects of incontinence. In *Incontinence and its Management* (Mandelstam D., ed.) London: Croom Helm.
International Continence Society (1976). First report on the standardization of terminology of lower urinary tract function. *British Journal of Urology*, 48, 39–42.
Judd M. (1989). *Mobility: Patient Problems and Nursing Care.* Oxford: Heinemann Nursing.
Menninger K. A. (1941). Some observations on the psychological factors in urination and genito-urinary afflictions. *Psychoanalytic Review*, 281, 117–29.
Palmtag H., Reidasch G. (1980). Psychogenic voiding patterns. *Urologia Internationalis*, 35, 321–7.
Schwartz M. S., Stanton A. H. (1950). A social psychological study of incontinence. *Psychiatry*, 13, 299–327.
Stanton S. L. (1984). *Clinical Gynaecology – Gynaecological Urology.* St Louis: C. V. Mosby.
Yarnell J. W. G., Volye G. J., Sweetnam P. M. et al (1982). Factors associated with urinary incontinence in women. *Journal of Epidemiology and Community Health*, 36, 58–63.

Bibliography

Booth J. A. (1983). *Handbook of Investigations.* London: Harper & Row.
Brocklehurst J. C. (1978). *The Genito-Urinary System. Textbook of*

Geriatric Medicine and Gerontology, 2nd edn. Edinburgh: Churchill Livingstone.

Charlton C. A. V. (1984). *The Urological System*. Edinburgh: Churchill Livingstone.

Freeman R. (1987). Open to suggestion. *Nursing Times*, **83** (46), 68–73.

Griffiths D. J. (1980). *Urodynamics: The Mechanism and Hydrodynamics of Incontinence of the Lower Urinary Tract*. Bristol: Adam Hilgar.

3

Patient assessment

INTRODUCTION

Assessment may involve a number of different disciplines, such as medicine, nursing, physiotherapy, occupational therapy, and radiology. It is therefore important that those involved in assessment are aware of each other's role. Such awareness may prevent the repetition of questions and investigations, thus reducing the risk of embarrassment or annoyance to the patient.

The aim of this text is to provide a nursing focus, based on a model of self-care.

NURSING MODELS

Nursing practice is constantly evolving as nurses endeavour to meet the changing demands society makes on the profession. In the last two decades nursing models have been created; these form a logical framework on which to base nursing interventions and actions. Some of these models have received wide acclaim, others much less so. The model of nursing used in this text is based on work described by Dorothea Orem (1985) in which she emphasizes the philosophy of self-care.

SELF-CARE

Orem's self-care model is concerned with the ability of individuals to maintain a delicate balance between their self-care abilities and the demands made upon them. In everyday life Orem suggests than an individual needs sufficient self-care ability to meet six universal self-care demands:

1 Sufficient intake of air, food and water.
2 Satisfactory eliminatory processes.
3 Maintaining a balance between activity and rest.
4 Maintaining a balance between solitude and social interaction.
5 Prevention of danger or hazard to self.
6 Maintaining normalcy – being 'normal'.

In addition a person needs to be able to practise self-care to meet developmental demands throughout life and must also have the necessary self-care ability to cope with illness.

Some may experience limitations in their own self-care ability or have additional needs due to changes in their physical, psychological or social circumstances. These changes may be through illness, injury or disease and may leave the individual unable to meet the necessary demands to maintain self-care. This may then result in a deficit between health care demand and self-care ability. When such a situation arises, nursing intervention would be required if the individual or his or her relative or significant other is unable to maintain a balance between demand and need.

JUSTIFICATION FOR NURSING INTERVENTION

In assessing the patient using Orem's model we therefore have to determine what demands are being made upon the individual to practise self-care and what abilities are required to meet those demands. If the patient's ability meets the demand, and looks as though it will continue to do so in the future, then no patient problem is said to exist.

However, if there is a deficit in self-care, whether now or potential, then there is a patient problem and nursing intervention is required. Nursing intervention can consist of carrying out the task entirely for the patient; assisting the patient; giving guidance or teaching the patient to practise self-care (Pearson and Vaughan, 1986).

Consider the following case history, bearing in mind Orem's ideas about self-care and nursing.

CASE HISTORY: MR CHARLES

Mr Charles was 76 years old and had been living with his daughter, son-in-law and two grandchildren since his wife died 4 years ago. He was admitted to hospital for 2 weeks' holiday relief whilst his daughter and family went away. On admission he appeared to the admitting nurse to be extremely agitated. As the nurse began to question Mr Charles, his daughter interjected and said that he was very worried about coming into hospital because he suffered from a 'lack of control over his bowels and bladder'. Mr Charles was immediately reassured by the nurse that the staff on the ward would do everything to make his stay as comfortable as possible, and do their best to sort out the problems he was having with his bowels and bladder.

He appeared mentally alert, although obviously distressed by his symptoms. During the discussion which followed he revealed that up until 6 months ago he had been relatively healthy, and had led quite an active life. He loved walking and took the family dog for a walk each day; he also enjoyed gardening and going out, often accompanying his son-in-law to the local pub for a drink. Then suddenly he had developed a cold, which led to a chest infection, causing him to take to his bed for about 2 weeks. The local general practitioner was called and prescribed medication for the infection.

Mr Charles said he had never regained his former fitness, his appetite was still quite poor and he had little energy to do anything other than get up and get dressed. He had noticed that his bowel motions had tended to become irregular and for the past 3 months he found he frequently soiled himself as he had insufficient time to get to the toilet when he felt the urge – it was often only seconds before his bowels acted. He had also noticed that his urine had become much darker in colour and gave off a very unpleasant odour; he went several times a day to the toilet, but on occasions only passed small amounts; sometimes he found he had wet himself before he could get there.

The soiling of his clothing and bedding caused him great

embarrassment, and also distress at the extra work this created for his daughter.

Mr Charles's daughter was very understanding of her father, but admitted that she was beginning to feel a little embarrassed when friends called unexpectedly at the house and she had not had a chance to remove her father's 'special chair' out of the lounge. (The chair was well padded and protected, at the insistence of Mr Charles.) She also found the soiled undergarments rather distasteful and would often resort to throwing them away rather than have them soaking in a bucket, especially at weekends when the children were home or if they were entertaining friends.

Neither Mr Charles nor his daughter had considered contacting the general practitioner about the loss of control over his bladder and bowel function. The nurse carrying out the assessment felt that it was almost as if they viewed the situation as inevitable with advancing age.

We shall continue with Mr Charles's case later; meanwhile, consider what additional information might be required and what initial investigation should be undertaken to try and identify the cause of these symptoms.

ESSENTIAL ATTRIBUTES WHEN UNDERTAKING A NURSING ASSESSMENT

For a nursing assessment to be meaningful to both nurse and patient, the nurse must possess certain skills and qualities. These skills are even more important when trying to obtain information which may be potentially embarrassing to the patient, especially if he or she has gone to great lengths to conceal the problem from relatives or friends, as is often the case when a person is incontinent.

A nurse should therefore demonstrate the ability to:

1 Use effective questioning techniques.
2 Listen carefully to what the patient says.
3 Appear attentive during the assessment.
4 Reflect on and clarify issues raised by the patient.
5 Use pauses and silence to advantage.

6 Observe the patient accurately.
7 Observe the patient's responses to his or her environment.

In carrying out the assessment the nurse needs to be:

1 Tactful at all times.
2 Non-judgemental.
3 Approachable.
4 Able to create an atmosphere based on mutual trust and respect.

QUESTIONS

Nurses spend a large proportion of their time asking questions, but often for no clearly defined purpose. It is important, particularly when dealing with a distressing symptom like incontinence, that the nurse has a clear understanding of the following:

1 What information is required?
2 Why is it required?
3 When is it required by?
4 How is it to be obtained?
5 Where is the most appropriate source to obtain that information?
6 Who is going to obtain the information?
7 What is to happen to the information, once obtained?

Such clarity can avoid duplication of questions, minimizing embarrassment to the patient. It is equally important for the patient to be viewed as a whole person, not reduced to a symptomatic approach. Hence the value of nursing models like Orem's, which provide a humanistic and holistic approach on which to base nursing intervention.

HISTORY

If continence is to be restored, or incontinence to be more effectively managed, it is essential to begin with an accurate history of the patient. The importance of good interview technique has been stressed, as has the need for a clear understanding of the information required and the reasons why.

Ideally, at least part of the assessment should be conducted in the patient's usual environment. This enables the assessor to observe if any factors in the environment may be causing or influencing the incontinence; also, the patient may feel more relaxed at home and be more willing to discuss incontinence. This may not always be the case, especially when the symptom has been or is being concealed from other members of the family. The person conducting the assessment must therefore be sensitive to each situation and act in a manner which will promote the patient's confidence and co-operation.

The first hurdle to overcome is getting the patient to talk frankly about the situation and its effects. In the majority of cases, it is the doctor and nurse who are initially involved in the assessment. Ideally a medical and nursing assessment should be carried out simultaneously to avoid the risk of duplicating questions (see Figs. 3.1 and 3.2).

Recording patient information

Modern technology has made available a variety of methods for recording and storing patient information. However, the most commonly used method within the health care professions is still a hand-written record. Each discipline appears to have its own format and variation within the same discipline is not uncommon. Despite this wide variation in format, most records contain similar biographical details. It is essential to ensure that relevant information is available to others involved in the patient's care to avoid repetitive questioning.

Problems of recording information

Some professional carers experience problems of recording information when using pre-printed history and assessment forms. A common problem is a lack of space under an appropriate heading. Whilst such difficulties can easily be overcome by simple adaptation, many people solve the

Nursing Assessment of an Incontinent Patient

Incontinence is always a *symptom* of an underlying problem, never a problem in itself.

Definition of continence

To recognise the need to empty the bladder or bowel.

To "hold on" until it is convenient to go.

Being able to recognise and get to a toilet.

Being able to undress.

Being able to use a toilet.

History

Listen carefully – take time.

GENERAL INFORMATION

Name, address, date of birth

Family, number of children.

Others living in the home.

Facilities in the home – how many and where are the toilets?

Are there any other toileting aids, commodes, urinals etc?

GENERAL MEDICAL HISTORY

Any operations, past illnesses, medication. Mental state, mobility, dexterity?

SPECIFIC HISTORY OF INCONTINENCE

Patient's attitude to the problem.

Carer's attitude to the problem.

When did incontinence start?

Is it associated with an event in the past or present?

Are there any pads, pants etc. used at present? If so which type?

DAY

- How often is urine passed normally?
- When do episodes of leakage occur?
- How much?
- Is there leakage on coughing, sneezing, physical exertion?
- Can the patient hold on, or do they have to get to a toilet quickly?
- Is the stream good?
- Is the patient aware of leakage?
- Does the patient dribble after passing urine?

NIGHT

- Does the patient have to get up at night?
- How many times?
- Is the patient incontinent?

FLUID INTAKE, BOWEL HABITS, DIET

PHYSICAL EXAMINATION

Abdominal – palpable bladder/large bowel.

Urethra, Perineum, Vagina, Urethritis, Vaginitis, Leakage on coughing.

Residual urine.

Rectal examination, constipation.

URINE TEST

Routine urine test, mid-stream specimen.

BASE LINE CHART

INDIVIDUAL CARE PLAN

SET REALISTIC OBJECTIVES

Treatment

Adjustment of facilities and clothing, retraining, toileting plan from Base Chart.

Medication used in conjunction with toileting plan.

Pelvic floor exercises, correct aids.

Adjustment of bowel habits.

Diet and fluid adaption.

Remember

Everyone is different, anxiety exacerbates the problem, privacy, home assessment is more realistic, many patients can become continent, incontinence can be managed with dignity. Do we encourage incontinence by spending more time with incontinent patients?

This Assessment Form was designed by Hilary Oliver, Nurse Continence Advisor, General Hospital, Nottingham. © HGW Ltd 1987.

Fig. 3.1. *Nursing assessment form of an incontinent patient. Reproduced by kind permission.*

Patient's name _____ Hospital _____
Address _____
GP _____

Patient's name _____ Hospital _____
Ward _____
Consultant _____

1 Is the patient incontinent

Yes | 1
No | 0

If yes answer all questions
If no continue at question 6

2 Is the patient incontinent of

Urine | 1
Faces | 1
Both | 3

3 How often is the patient incontinent

1 – 2 x daily | 1
2 – 5 x daily | 2
More than 5 times | 3

4 Is the patient incontinent during

Day | 1
Night | 2
Both | 3

5 How long has the patient been incontinent

Under 1 month | 1
1 – 6 months | 2
6 – 12 months | 3
Over a year | 4

6 Does the patients have a catheter

Yes | 1
No | 0

7 Is the patient

Ambulant | 1
Able to stand with help | 2
Unable to stand | 3

8 Is the patient

Mentally alert | 1
Slightly confused | 2
Very confused | 3

9 Does the patient take diuretics

Yes | 1
No | 0

10 Is the patient aware of the problem

Yes | 0
No | 1

11 Is the patient

Male | 1
Female | 2

12 Is the patient's skin condition

Good | 1
Red | 2
Broken | 3

13 How long has the patient been in hospital

Under 1 month | 1
1–6 months | 2
6–12 months | 3
Over 1 year | 4

Patient's diagnosis

Patients total score

Guide to score results

Under 20 –
Good chance of becoming continent
Between 20 and 25 –
Fair chance of becoming continent
Over 25 –
Poor chance of becoming continent

Searby score chart

The Searby score chart has been designed to help nurses both within the community and hospital to easily identify their patients' incontinence problems. It is of a basic design and uses the same principles as the Norton Scale. The chart is easy to follow and depending on the patient's score you can determine whether or not continence is possible.

The scoring should take place with co-operation of the patient in privacy and the patient should not feel embarrassed about the questions asked. If the patient cannot answer the questions, the nurse should be able to use discretion and answer the questions on behalf of the patient.

By comparing the results of the score charts, you can monitor the patient's continence/incontinence. Ideally the charts should be completed monthly and compared to previous charts, thereby showing improvement or deterioration.

Fig. 3.1. *Continued.*

Nursing Incontinence Assessment Form

Date:

PATIENT DETAILS

Name...   Sex..

Address...   Tel no:..

Age...............Yrs   Occupation ....   No. of children..................................

GP name..   (if patient is female)

Referred by..   District nurse...................................

MEDICAL HISTORY Please give a brief description of patient's medical history relating to their incontinence including any investigations/surgery to date, drug treatment and any related conditions e.g. diabetes, arthritis
....
....

What were the circumstances at or reasons for the onset of the condition?
....
....

CURRENT CONDITION Please specify current symptoms and the clinical diagnosis associated with the patient's incontinence

Symptoms...

Diagnosis..

ADDITIONAL DETAILS

Weight...

Description of bowel function...

Volume of daily fluid intake..litres

Volume of daily urine output..litres

Specimen results: MSU... CSU..................................

	YES	NO	
Is the skin healthy	☐	☐	If no please describe...................
Is the vulva healthy	☐	☐	If not specify, e.g. vaginitis..............
Is blood present in the urine	☐	☐	
Is there burning or pain when passing urine	☐	☐	
Does the patients experience a sensation of fullness	☐	☐	
Is there incomplete emptying	☐	☐	
Is there a poor flow	☐	☐	
Is there any hesitancy	☐	☐	
Does suprapubic pressure improve the flow	☐	☐	
Is this used regularly	☐	☐	

CONTINENCE DETAILS Please delete as necessary

Is the leak continuous.. Yes/No

Is the urine loss.. A dribble/A fair stream/The entire contents

Does incontinence occur.. Day and night/Mostly at night/Mostly during the day

Is the patient aware of dribbling............................... Yes/No/Sometimes

Is the patient wet when sitting .... Yes/No/Sometimes

Does the patient wet the bed.................................... Yes/No/Sometimes

Does the patient dribble after passing water........... Yes/No   (continued)

Fig. 3.2. *A Squibb Surgicare Ltd nursing incontinence assessment form. Reproduced by kind permission.*

Do any of the following precipitate incontinence?   Please tick as necessary

Walking   □
Coughing/laughing/other physical strain   □
Change of position   □
Anxiety/fear   □
Urgency   □
Does the condition ever vary? Yes/No. If yes, reasons if any..
Is the condition . . . improving/the same/worsening

TOILETTING

How many times does the patient visit a toilet: In the day......................times
                                                     At night........................times

Does the patient visit the toilet: Can the patient hold on once there is a need to
             Please tick   pass water. Please tick

Only when there is a desire to go   □   For: Less than one minute   □
Hourly   □   1 – 2 minutes   □
2-hourly   □   2 – 5 minutes   □
4-hourly   □   5 – 10 minutes   □
On some other regular basis   □   Longer   □

HOME/SOCIAL CIRCUMSTANCES

Please specify: Location of toilet/s...
                    Degree of dexterity..
                    Any restrictions of mobility...
                    Any eyesight limitations..
                    Any problems with washing/dressing/hygiene.....................
                    Any problems getting to/on toilet.......................................
Does patient do own shopping...
Does incontinence interfere with social activities...
Is patient's attitude to the problem . . . distressed/unconcerned/other.................

TREATMENT

Incontinence aids used at present...
Incontinence aids obtained from...
How much per week does patient spend on them..

ACTION THIS VISIT

Details of supplies given...
Supplies obtained from/through..
Arrangements/communication with GP..
Details of any hospital referral...

INVESTIGATIONS THIS VISIT (Please tick as appropriate)

MSU   □   CSU   □   Pelvic floor tone □
Skin condition □   Rectal examination   □   PV examination   □
Bowels   □   Residual urine   □   Other   □

FUTURE RECOMMENDATIONS

Details of home visits...
Details of clinic appointment..
Details of hospital admission...

Fig. 3.2.   Continued.

problem by limiting the information they record. This is particularly noticeable under headings such as elimination when the patient is known to be incontinent. Instead of information about the person's elimination pattern being recorded, one frequently finds the word 'incontinent' written without further explanation.

Checklists

Over the years a number of checklists have been developed for use as an aide-mémoire to obtain more detailed information about a person's incontinence. When skilfully used, these checklists provide a useful and logical framework for eliciting and recording information. Unfortunately, not everyone appears to be aware how to use this type of aid; the result is that the checklist is sometimes used as a questionnaire with every question asked, regardless of its relevance to the person being assessed. The Disabled Living Foundation provides useful checklists and guidelines for professionals on urinary and faecal incontinence. Examples of different types of checklists are given at the end of this chapter.

MEDICAL EXAMINATION

Everyone who presents with incontinence should have a full medical examination if the causes of the incontinence are to be established and appropriate treatment instigated. This will include investigation and assessment of the patient's general physical state. If the patient's mental state is considered to be a causal factor, then a simple questionnaire to assess mental status can be administered. An example of the type of questions asked and the method of scoring is given in Fig. 3.3.

The physical examination will include careful palpation of the patient's abdomen for signs of bladder distension or other abnormality and a digital rectal examination to assess constipation, prostatic enlargement, rectal prolapse or tumour. Inspection of the vulval area will reveal signs of skin excoriation, congenital abnormalities or vaginitis. It is also possible to observe bulging of the introitus and leakage of urine when the patient with stress incontinence coughs. A vaginal examination will indicate the position of the cervix and condition of the vaginal walls. The strength of the patient's pelvic floor muscles and ability to tighten the vagina can be assessed by placing two fingers in the vagina and asking the patient to tighten the pelvic floor muscles.

ASSESSMENT OF SELF-CARE REQUIREMENTS

As observed before (p. 40), a person may experience limitations in his or her self-care ability or have additional self-care needs. Assessment of an individual's self-care ability helps to provide a baseline from which to monitor that person's progress. In addition it can indicate areas where intervention by others is required and may also assist in the diagnosis of current or potential problems.

The following assessment criteria are based on Orem's (1985) universal self-care needs (see p. 39). The information elicited under each of the six headings is similar to that which you may obtain from patients presenting with various types of incontinence.

Sufficient intake of air, food and water

The distress of incontinence can result in individuals or their relatives and carers deliberately restricting fluid intake in an

	Score
1 Today's date	0 or 1
2 Day of the week	0 or 1
3 Present address	0 or 1
4 Year born	0 or 1
5 Place of birth	0 or 1
6 Count backwards from 20 to 1 (correctly)	0 or 1
7 Name of the present month	0 or 1
8 Name of the present prime minister	0 or 1
9 Events during past 3 months (in sequence)	0 or 1
10 Name of next of kin	0 or 1

Score of 7 out of 10 = borderline.

Fig. 3.3. *Mental status questionnaire.*

attempt to promote continence. Alternatively, some people may be unable through physical or mental deficit to obtain or consume sufficient fluid. Certain types of beverages, like tea, coffee and cola, which contain caffeine or alcohol can precipitate incontinence and are best avoided or taken in small quantities.

An important aspect of assessment is to determine what the patient drinks; how much, and when. Similar information is also required about the individual's dietary habits as factors such as roughage content will affect eliminatory function. If a patient is found to have a self-care deficit in food or fluid intake the nurse should attempt to determine the reasons why, and assess the probability of the patient re-establishing self-care needs.

Satisfactory eliminatory process

Whenever incontinence exists elimination ceases to be a satisfactory function for the individual concerned.

Defecation

Bowel habits vary considerably and may be influenced by physical, psychological, social, economic and cultural factors, yet most can be classified as normal. The average patterns of defecation for adults in the UK range from three times a day to once every 3 days (Connell et al, 1965). There can be few symptoms that cause the distress associated with faecal incontinence, or which require the nurse to demonstrate such a high degree of interpersonal skill. For ease of reference the causes of faecal incontinence can be categorized under three main headings – faecal impaction, colonic and anorectal disorders and neurological damage.

Micturition

Unsatisfactory patterns of voiding may arise for a variety of reasons, as indicated in Chapter 2, and with varying degrees of severity. Some people may experience difficulty in commencing urine flow; alternatively dribbling may be the problem, either constantly or following cessation of a main stream. The latter may be due to urine becoming trapped in the bulbar urethra and slowly being released later, whereas continuous dribbling is usually a result of damage to the urethral sphincters or if the sphincters are inactive or incomplete due to trauma, congenital lesion or nerve damage. Dysuria is the term used to define a painful burning sensation often felt during voiding which is commonly associated with urinary tract infection or atrophic urethritis.

Strangury

Some patients complain of severe pain radiating down the shaft of the penis to the urethral meatus. This symptom is associated with bladder distension due to obstruction from a blood clot or stone. Frequency of micturition is a common urinary symptom and is said to be present if a person has to void seven or more times during the day. Causes of frequency include obstruction or narrowing of the urethra, neurogenic bladder, excessive production of urine (polyuria), small bladder syndrome or bladder infection (cystitis).

Hesitancy

This refers to a situation that arises when a person consciously wants to void and is in the appropriate place and position, but experiences a delay in initiating the flow. This may occur if the desire to void has been deliberately suppressed over a period of time, causing the bladder to distend, or if the bladder outlet or urethra is obstructed. Hesitancy is quite common in men who have an enlargement of the prostate gland.

Nocturia

Most people, once in bed and asleep, are rarely woken by the conscious desire to micturate. Nocturia is the term used when referring to a minority of people who are woken by the need to void. It is, however, important for the nurse to ascertain that the patient was woken by this desire, and had not wakened for some other reason and then decided to micturate.

Sometimes nocturia results from an obsession to void frequently; alternatively the cause could be the consumption of large quantities of fluid late in the evening, or inappropriate timing of medication such as diuretics. Patients with cystitis or atrophic vaginitis frequently complain of nocturia; many elderly people suffer from this symptom due to a loss of normal diurnal variation. Robinson and Brocklehurst (1986) reported the appearance of atrophic changes in the vaginal mucosa of elderly patients referred with incontinence.

Bed-wetting can occur at any age and for a variety of reasons. In some instances the patient may be awake but unaware of the need to void; others may be both awake and aware, but lack the necessary control, dexterity, mobility or co-ordination to maintain continence. The term nocturnal enuresis is used to describe voiding whilst asleep, and is usually associated with children and young adults in the absence of organic causes such as infection or obstruction. Drugs – particularly sedatives – can also result in some people voiding whilst sleeping. It is therefore important during assessment to ask the patient about medication.

Stress incontinence is the term used to describe an involuntary leakage of urine. This symptom may be mild or severe and is more common amongst women. It usually occurs when lifting, coughing, sneezing or undertaking any activity which increases intra-abdominal pressure, causing the pressure in the bladder to become greater than that in the urethra, thus allowing leakage to occur. The patient may also have a weak or incompetent urethral sphincter mechanism or neurogenic bladder. A person with stress incontinence may, if the symptom is mild, complain of dampness of undergarments or in severe cases, of being soaked through to top clothes.

Urgency and urge incontinence

The time interval between the conscious desire to micturate and the uncontrollable urge to void is normally at least an hour. However, some people only have a new moments between the desire to void and the act of voiding; this symptom is referred to as urgency. If the patient is unable to find a suitable place to void, this can result in urge incontinence. This type of incontinence is associated with conditions like cystitis or bladder instability.

Maintaining a balance between activity and rest

Nocturia can severely restrict the amount of sleep an individual has, to the extent that an imbalance between rest and activity may develop. Frequency can increase the level of activity required by a person beyond what he or she is capable of. Alternatively incontinence may lead to a person being too embarrassed to go out at all. A self-care deficit in activity can be *caused by* incontinence as well as being the *cause of* incontinence (Judd, 1989).

Many people experience great difficulty in getting to or from the toilet. Factors such as how many steps have to be negotiated to reach the toilet should be considered. For others, adjusting clothing or sitting down and getting up from the toilet seat are also problematic.

During assessment of mobility the feet and type of footwear worn should be examined to exclude common causes of limited mobility like callouses, long toenails, ill-fitting shoes, and excessive use of slippers, to name but a few.

Maintaining a balance between solitude and social interaction

Many incontinent people become increasingly isolated. This may be a voluntary decision, or enforced by the actions of others. One of the main reasons for the curtailment of social interaction is the risk of accidents and the embarrassment this may cause to the sufferer and those in attendance. The person is afraid that the unmistakable odour from soiled undergarments may permeate the atmosphere and be detected by others. If aids are worn to contain the incontinence, the wearer may be concerned about detection by others and this may inhibit social activity.

Social isolation can lead to impaired mental function due to lack of stimulation. Boredom, a loss of contact with reality and confusion can all start to develop from social isolation. It is not always easy for the nurse to assess the extent and effect of a person's solitude on social interaction and considerable tact and skill are required to elicit this type of information.

Prevention of danger or hazard to self

There are many dangers and hazards facing individuals in their daily lives. Normally we practise self-care and avoid them, but incontinence exposes individuals to significant hazards that would otherwise be avoided. An example is the risk of dehydration due to inadequate fluid intake.

Incontinence can increase the risk of accidents at home or at work if the individual is rushing to the toilet. The risk is even greater when the person has defective eyesight and is in an unfamiliar environment.

Skin excoriation and infection are both potential hazards if the ability to maintain personal hygiene becomes impaired due to incontinence. Soiling of undergarments and the inability to wipe oneself properly following elimination increase this risk.

Maintaining normalcy

For the vast majority of people who have incontinence, this means giving up many activities they had previously undertaken, and, at worst, ceasing to lead 'normal' lives. Mr Charles's case history (p. 40) gives a clear indication of the effects that incontinence may have on normalcy. Increased family tension, disharmony, the inability to function effectively in one's everyday capacity, and withdrawal from sexual relationships are just a few examples of how normal lives may be disrupted.

INVESTIGATION OF INCONTINENCE

Incontinence may be due to more than one primary source, therefore the assessment procedure should include various tests if it is to be comprehensive. However, it is equally important not to subject the patient to a range of tests unnecessarily. If the initial history is obtained through detailed observation and interview then the appropriateness of any tests should be explained to the patient.

Urinalysis

All nurses are familiar with urinalysis and its importance in aiding diagnosis. The most commonly used testing agents are the reagent sticks which are dipped in the urine and read in accordance with the manufacturers' instructions. Routine investigation usually includes observation of urine colour. In health, urine is generally transparent and amber-coloured. It may become darker when concentrated, or very pale when diluted. The colour of urine may be affected by certain drugs or other chemical reactions within the body. The laxative Dorbanex, for example, tends to make urine red, as does eating beetroot. The injection of certain dyes for the purpose of radiological examination gives a blue-green appearance to the urine. Urobilogen tends to darken the urine quite considerably. The appearance of blood (haematuria) is usually unmistakable.

If the urine has a cloudy appearance this may be due to the presence of pus cells or debris and requires the testing of an early morning mid-stream specimen of urine (EMSU) in order to identify the presence of micro-organisms. The patient is asked to wash the genital area, then collect in a sterile container the middle portion of the first urine specimen made on rising that morning. (The greatest concentration of organisms is usually present in the first morning specimen.)

Cytology examination may be indicated when tumour formation is suspected. This requires a fresh specimen of urine to be obtained and then centrifuged. The deposits are stained and slides made for the pathologist to examine.

The value of having an accurate record of the amount and times a patient voids over each 24-hour period cannot be over-estimated. Yet what may appear to be a simple task is often the most difficult to achieve with any degree of satisfaction, due mainly to the nurse or patient forgetting to measure accurately and record the information.

Charts

There are several different types of charts available for recording information about the amount, type and time a patient voids. Some are very simple to use; others are more sophisticated. It is therefore important to select the appropriate type of chart. The following questions should be asked.

1 What information is required, and for what purpose?
2 Who is to fill in the chart, and where is it to be used? (Professional carer, patient, relative, a combination of people; for use in hospital or at home or both.)
3 Are there any factors which will inhibit use of the chart? (Lack of time or motivation by professional carers, problems of dexterity, impairment of patient's mental function, amount of information required, lack of motivation or understanding on the part of the patient or family.)

It is always a good idea when contemplating the use of charts to tell those involved with the recording of information how long the record is to be kept for. In most situations sufficient information should be obtained within 1 or 2 weeks. Furthermore the majority of people do not mind making an extra effort to do something if they know it is not for an indefinite period, and understand the value of the investigation. The two main reasons for using such charts are to provide a more accurate assessment of the patient's voiding pattern, and to enable a programme of treatment to be monitored more effectively. Charts are not an end in themselves but act as a record which can be interpreted in the light of all the other findings of the assessment (Norton, 1986).

The majority of charts comprise the days of the week and the hours of the day. In addition, space to record specific instructions is usually available (Fig. 3.4). Some charts give a list of codes to be used – W = wet; D = dry; PU = passed urine; NPU = not passed urine. Others may ask if the patient asked to use the toilet, or whether he or she was offered the opportunity (Fig. 3.5).

Disadvantages of charts

The advantages of using charts generally outweigh any disadvantages. However, much can still be done to improve unsatisfactory aspects. Space sometimes precludes all the relevant information being recorded, or results in the chart

Chart

Week commencing_____ Name_____

| Please tick in left-hand column each time urine is passed |
| Please tick in right-hand column each time you are wet |

Special instructions_____

_____

_____

	Monday		Tuesday		Wednesday		Thursday		Friday		Saturday		Sunday	
6 a.m.														
7 a.m.														
8 a.m.														
9 a.m.														
10 a.m.														
11 a.m.														
12 p.m.														
1 p.m.														
2 p.m.														
3 p.m.														
4 p.m.														
5 p.m.														
6 p.m.														
7 p.m.														
8 p.m.														
9 p.m.														
10 p.m.														
11 p.m.														
12 a.m.														
1 a.m.														
2 a.m.														
3 a.m.														
4 a.m.														
5 a.m.														
Totals														

Fig. 3.4. *Sample chart to record patient voiding.*

Promotion of Continence Chart

Instructions: **Make an entry in the chart each time the patient passes urine, has a bowel movement or is incontinent, by recording the code letters in the space for that day and hour.**

PU Passes urine (normally)
PF Passes faeces (normally)
BW Bed wet
BS Bed soiled (faeces)
C   Commode

CS Clothes soiled (faeces)
R   Requested by patient
T   Toilet
CW Clothes wet
B   Bottle

Name:		*Ward:*			*Week commencing:*		
Time	**Monday**	**Tuesday**	**Wednesday**	**Thursday**	**Friday**	**Saturday**	**Sunday**
8 a.m.							
9 a.m.							
10 a.m.							
11 a.m.							
Midday							
1 p.m.							
2 p.m.							
3 p.m.							
4 p.m.							
5 p.m.							
6 p.m.							
7 p.m.							
8 p.m.							
9 p.m.							
10 p.m.							
11 p.m.							
Midnight							
1 a.m.							
2 a.m.							
3 a.m.							
4 a.m.							
5 a.m.							
6 a.m.							
7 a.m.							

Fig. 3.5. *Promotion of continence chart.*

being untidy and difficult to read. Often ticks are used to denote urine passed in an appropriate receptacle and/or episodes of incontinence without any indication of the volume passed. (Sometimes it is sufficient just to indicate frequency.) Charts with times printed on them may already have a negative influence on both patient and carer, as they may feel something *ought* to be recorded every hour regardless. Complicated or lengthy instructions can cause confusion to the user, as can the use of too many abbreviations or complicated colour coding. Some people tend not to fill in the chart as and when the information becomes available, which may result in the information being forgotten and hence not recorded.

Examples of how charting can aid diagnosis

The information depicted by the three continence charts shown in Figs. 3.6–3.8 is typical of three common bladder symptoms. Study each one and try to decide what symptom each chart is highlighting.

Having discussed the nursing assessment of the patient, it remains to describe briefly some of the medical investigations that may be carried out.

MEDICAL INVESTIGATIONS

Blood tests

Blood tests are prescribed as part of a urological investigation for various reasons. A standard cell count and electrolyte analysis will help to determine the patient's general health status. Red cell production may be depressed due to uraemia, causing anaemia to develop, while if the patient has oliguria (diminished urine secretion), then this may give rise to an increase in serum potassium and the condition of hyperkalaemia, which can seriously affect the body's neuromuscular function. The serum levels of bicarbonate, sodium and chloride can also be drastically affected by changes in the body's fluid content or distribution.

If renal calculi are suspected, then measurement of the levels of serum calcium and uric acid will assist the diagnosis. Blood urea and creatinine levels measure renal function while a raised level of the enzyme acid phosphatase assists in confirming cancer of the prostate gland.

Radiological investigation

A straight abdominal x-ray will show any radiopaque calculus or areas of calcification within the urinary tract. It may also be possible to assess the contours of the kidney and evaluate bladder size by close scrutiny of soft tissue shadow. Findings from the straight abdominal x-ray combined with information of the patient's history may indicate to the medical staff the need for an intravenous pyelogram (IVP) or intravenous urogram (IVU). A contrast medium is injected into the patient's vein whilst an image intensifier monitors its flow through the veins to the excretory organs. Radiographs are taken as the dye is excreted via the kidneys (pyelogram) and at various intervals throughout its passage along the urinary tract (urogram). A radiograph is usually taken after excretion of the dye to ascertain if the patient has any residual urine.

A retrograde pyelogram or ascending examination may be required if the IVP/IVU findings indicate evidence of a tumour, calculi, malfunctioning kidney or urethral stricture. A contrast medium is injected into the ureters under aseptic conditions via a small-bore ureteric catheter. The catheter is usually introduced following cystoscopy. This procedure is mainly done with the patient anaesthetized.

Micturating cystourethrogram is an x-ray examination of the bladder and urethra following the introduction of a contrast medium via a urethral catheter into the bladder. X-rays are then taken with the patient at rest, straining but without voiding, and after removal of the catheter with the patient voiding. The findings can indicate the presence of vesicoureteric reflux.

Cystoscopy

A cystoscope is used to examine the bladder by direct vision. This type of examination will require the patient to be

Chart

Week commencing _7th October_ Name _Mrs Davidson_

Special instructions _____

Please measure and record amount of urine

passed.

	Monday		Tuesday		Wednesday		Thursday		Friday		Saturday		Sunday	
6 a.m.														
7 a.m.	450		400		400		350		400					
8 a.m.											350		400	
9 a.m.	150	W	200							W				
10 a.m.				W	250		200	W	300				150	
11 a.m.					100	W					200	W		
12 p.m.			250											
1 p.m.	300						250		200	W			250	
2 p.m.					150	W					250			
3 p.m.														
4 p.m.	200	W	300	W			250		150				200	
5 p.m.					300			W					100	
6 p.m.							100				200			
7 p.m.	150		200						200					W
8 p.m.					250									
9 p.m.						W	250				300		200	
10 p.m.	300													
11 p.m.			300		200				350				250	
12 a.m.	100		100				250				200			
1 a.m.														
2 a.m.														
3 a.m.														
4 a.m.														
5 a.m.														
Totals	1650		1750		1650		1650		1550		1500		1550	

Fig. 3.6.   *Sample chart to record patient voiding.*

Chart

Week commencing __7th October__ Name __Mr Jackson__

Special instructions_____

__Please measure and record amount of urine__
__passed.__

	Monday	Tuesday	Wednesday	Thursday	Friday	Saturday	Sunday
6 a.m.	150		150			100	50
7 a.m.	30	100	50	100	50	50	90
8 a.m.		80		30		30	
9 a.m.	80		90		70		70
10 a.m.	100	120	70	60	30	60	30
11 a.m.	50	40		50		40	60
12 p.m.			40	30	40		
1 p.m.	90	50	60		30		50
2 p.m.	40	30	50	90		70	40
3 p.m.	60	40				50	
4 p.m.			30	50	70	30	
5 p.m.	80	100			10		100
6 p.m.	60	50	70	80	50	40	
7 p.m.	50		40	40	80		
8 p.m.		60				60	90
9 p.m.	100	40	120		60	90	
10 p.m.			40	100		50	40
11 p.m.	120	90		40	100		50
12 a.m.		50	90		70	90	
1 a.m.			100				
2 a.m.	150 W			50 W	40 W		100
3 a.m.		100				100 W	
4 a.m.	60 W		50				
5 a.m.				60			
Totals	1220	950	1050	780	700	860	770

Fig. 3.7. *Sample chart to record patient voiding.*

Chart

Week commencing __7ᵗʰ October__ Name __Mrs Mason__

Special instructions_____

Please try to measure and record amount of
urine passed

	Monday		Tuesday		Wednesday		Thursday		Friday		Saturday		Sunday	
6 a.m.					120				150					
7 a.m.	150		200				200						200	
8 a.m.					100				120		200			
9 a.m.	80				50		100		60				90	
10 a.m.	100		150								120			
11 a.m.			40				90		100				150	
12 p.m.	60				150		60				90		100	W
1 p.m.	90		100	W										
2 p.m.					80		110	W	100		100		110	
3 p.m.	120	W			90						60			
4 p.m.			90						80	W			70	
5 p.m.			50				120				110		50	
6 p.m.	200				100				110					
7 p.m.			120										100	
8 p.m.	70				120		80				120			
9 p.m.									70					
10 p.m.	100		100				100				70		120	
11 p.m.	50				150				120					
12 a.m.											100		100	
1 a.m.			110											
2 a.m.							110							
3 a.m.	110	W							100		90	W		W
4 a.m.				W	120									
5 a.m.														
Totals	1130		960		1080		970		1010		1060		1090	

Fig. 3.8.   Sample chart to record patient voiding.

anaesthetized. The equipment has a powerful light attachment for good vision, and usually attachments for taking biopsy specimens and pictures. To avoid introducing infection into the bladder the technique is performed with sterile equipment and using an aseptic technique.

Urodynamic studies

Urodynamics is the term used to describe the technique of measuring pressure and flow in the lower urinary tract. This type of investigation includes the study of urine flow rates, cystometry video (bladder or intravesical measurement), cystourethrography (urethral pressure profile) and measurement of the intra-abdominal (rectal) pressure with radiography of the lower urinary tract. A permanent record of the flow rate, total bladder pressure, and detrusor pressure is obtained by a video recording plus sound commentary of the x-ray pictures.

Flow rate

There are various types of flow meters available (Figs 3.9 and 3.10). The rate of flow is calculated either by a weight transducer positioned under the collecting receptacle or by the urine passing on to a revolving disc placed inside the funnel of the commode seat. The energy required to turn the disc is calculated as the flow rate. The flow rate is expressed in millilitres per second; a normal pattern should resemble that found in Fig. 3.11 and Table 3.1. Note how the trace begins promptly and quickly reaches its peak, before swiftly dropping again and finishing promptly with no evidence of post-micturition dribbling. The flow rate should be at least 15 ml/s when an average of 200 ml of urine is passed.

Patients are asked to attend this investigation with a full bladder. The procedure is explained to the patient beforehand. The patient's privacy should be maintained throughout this non-invasive procedure. Even so, some patients, despite being able to micturate in private, find sitting or standing (usually on or over a commode-style seat), combined with the noise of urine hitting the receptacle, extremely embarrassing.

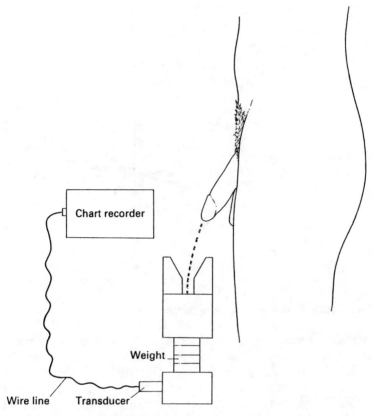

Fig. 3.9.   *Weight transducer flow meter. Men may prefer to stand; women may sit on a commode-style seat.*

Cystometry

Cystometry is possibly the most invasive investigation that a patient is subjected to. It should therefore only be used after a detailed history has been taken and a full medical examination and other appropriate investigations have been conducted and their findings assessed.

The investigation requires the patient to have two catheters in the bladder and a third in the rectum. One of the bladder catheters is used to fill the bladder, while the other records the total pressure within the bladder (intravesical pressure). The rectal catheter records the pressure within the rectum. Bladder

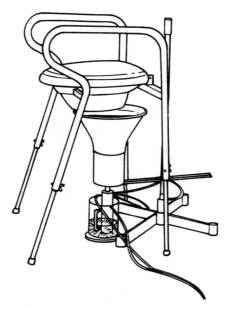

Fig. 3.10. *Rotating disc flow meter.*

pressure reflects both bladder activity as well as general pressure changes within the abdominal cavity. Therefore, if only total bladder pressure were recorded and measured, it would not give a true picture of detrusor activity. There is general agreement that the pressure within the rectum is equal to that of the intra-abdominal cavity, so if rectal pressure is subtracted from total bladder pressure, the remaining pressure reflects detrusor activity (detrusor pressure; see Fig. 3.12).

The full procedure should be carefully explained to the patient, using diagrams where appropriate. The nurse or doctor who is providing the explanation should allow plenty of time, and ensure the environment is conducive to a relaxed discussion. Always check the patient's understanding of the procedure before ending the interview and before commencing the investigation.

Procedure

The room where the patient is to have the investigation should be warm and designed in such a way as to ensure maximum

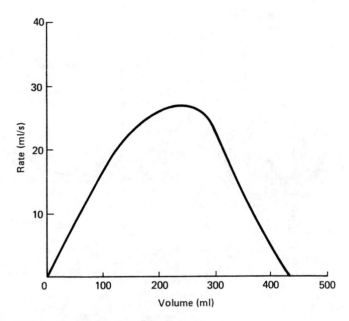

Fig. 3.11. *Normal urine flow rate.*

Table 3.1. Average voiding patterns

Age group	Rate
Males under 60	18–22 ml/s
Males over 60	13 ml/s
Females under 50	25–28 ml/s
Females over 50	18 ml/s

privacy. The patient should be asked to void urine; this may be into a flow meter. Afterwards the bladder should be catheterized and the residual urine measured and recorded together with any problems of catheterization. The filling catheter is then attached to the fluid reservoir (usually normal saline) via a giving set. The second catheter is connected to the pressure transducer to monitor the pressure. The rectal catheter is then passed and attached to the second pressure

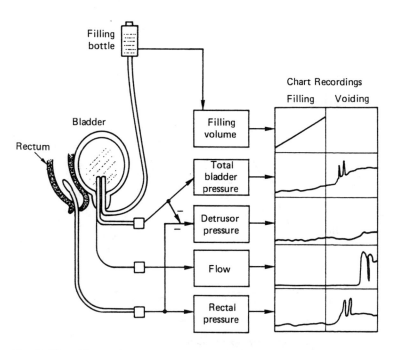

Fig. 3.12. *Normal cystometrogram information.*

transducer (see Fig. 3.12). The patient should be quietly reassured and kept informed throughout the procedure.

The bladder is quickly filled with fluid (approximately 100 ml/min) at room temperature. The patient should be lying in a supine position during the filling stage and asked to indicate when he or she has the first sensation of the desire to void; also when he or she feels that the bladder has reached maximum capacity without undue discomfort and whilst trying not to leak. During this period a chart recorder is providing a continuous read-out of the rectal, detrusor and bladder pressures. Normally, the detrusor pressure remains below the level of 15 cm water until voiding occurs; the first desire to void is usually experienced after the introduction of 150–200 ml of fluid, with the sensation of fullness occurring at bladder capacity of 350–600 ml. If leakage occurs this should be indicated on the recording.

When the subjective bladder capacity has been reached the filling catheter is removed and the patient is asked, and helped if necessary, to stand up, cough or jump up and down to demonstrate the competence of the sphincter. Any incontinence observed is recorded. The patient is then asked to void into a flow meter; normally the bladder will contract, creating a detrusor pressure of 40–60 cm water in men and 30–40 cm water in women.

Midway through voiding the patient is asked to try and interrupt the flow – this enables the closing mechanism of the urethra to be examined. The patient should be able rapidly to interrupt and recommence the flow on request, completely emptying the bladder.

The procedure takes approximately half an hour to complete, and is of major importance in the diagnosis of disorder of micturition.

Video cystourethrography

Many of the centres that provide facilities for urodynamic studies also have equipment to undertake video cystourethrography. This procedure differs from cystometry only in so far as the bladder is filled with a contrast medium (i.e. Dioclone), so as to allow visualization of the bladder and urethra. This technique is of value for patients who have had pelvic surgery, or where it is difficult to diagnose bladder or bladder neck abnormalities without direct vision.

Algorithmic method

Hilton and Stanton (1981) described an algorithmic method of assessing urinary incontinence in elderly women (Fig. 3.13).

Urethral pressure profile

Research on transducers to measure the intraurethral pressure is currently being evaluated. It is possible to insert a water-filled or microtransducer catheter into the bladder and then slowly withdraw it along the urethra to the external meatus whilst the pressure is being recorded by a chart recorder. This procedure is undertaken with the patient in a supine position.

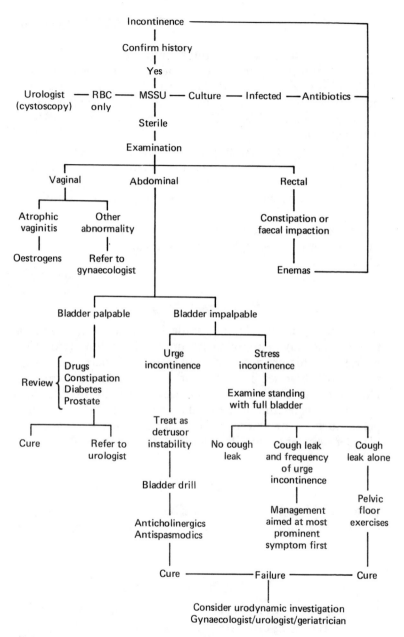

Fig. 3.13. *Algorithmic method of assessing urinary incontinence in elderly women. From Hilton and Stanton (1981), with permission. RBC = red blood cell count; MSSU = mid-stream specimen of urine.*

Electromyelography

The degree of striated muscle activity of the perianal or periurethral muscles can be measured either by directly placing a needle electrode into the muscle, or by a surface electrode. The information obtained can be helpful in determining reasons for urinary retention or incontinence and of faecal incontinence.

References

Connell A. M., Hilton C., Irvine G. et al (1965). Variation of bowel habit in two population samples. *British Medical Journal*, 11, 1095–9.
Hilton P., Stanton S. L. (1981). An algorithmic method for assessing urinary continence in elderly women. *British Medical Journal*, 282, 940–2.
Judd M. (1989). *Mobility: Patient Problems and Nursing Care.* Oxford: Heinemann Nursing.
Norton C. S. (1986). *Nursing for Continence.* Beaconsfield: Beaconsfield Publishers.
Orem D. (1985). *Nursing: Concepts of Practice* 3rd edn. New York: McGraw Hill.
Pearson A., Vaughan V. B. (1986). *Nursing Models for Practice.* Oxford: Heinemann.
Robinson J. M., Brocklehurst J. C. (1984). *Evaluation of Methods for Assessment of Bladder and Urethral Function: Urology in the Elderly.* London: Churchill Livingstone.

Bibliography

Bradbury S. M. (1988). *Collection of Urine Specimens in General Practice: to clean or not clean?*
Cromer M. J. (1981). *Ethical Issues in Health Care.* St Louis: C. V. Mosby.
Egan G. (1982). *The Skilled Helper.* Monterey, California: Brooks Cole.
Faulkner A. (1984). *Communication.* Edinburgh: Churchill Livingstone.
Gerrard B. A., Bonniface W. J., Lowe B. H. (1980). *Interpersonal Skills for Health Professionals.* Reston, Virginia: Reston.
Hamer L. M. (1985). *The Healthy Relationship: Process and Skills.* Englewood Cliffs, New Jersey: Prentice Hall.
Johnstone M. (1979). Anxiety/stress and the effects on disclosure

between nurses, patients. *Advances in Nursing Science*, 2, (4), 1–20.

Palmer J. H. (1982). Assessing and investigating urinary incontinence. *Geriatric Medicine*, 12, (1), 24–5.

Riehl J. P., Callister R. (1980). *Conceptual Models for Nursing Practice*. London: Appleton Century Croft.

Silverhurst J., Brown M., Shawer M. (1981). Assessing the severity of urinary incontinence in women by weighing a perineal pad. *Lancet*, May 23rd, 1, (8230), 1128–30.

Journal of the Royal College of Practitioners, 38, (313), 363–5.

Wessex Continence Advisers Association Learning Package (1986). For copies, please contact the Secretary, Wessex Continence Advisers Association.

4

Planning care

INTRODUCTION

The information obtained from the nursing history and assessment provides a framework for the design of the nursing intervention. Nursing, in relation to the model of self-care advocated in this text, may be defined as the giving of direct assistance to a person when he or she is unable to meet his or her own self-care needs. The requirements for nursing are modified and eventually eliminated when there is a progressive favourable change in the state of health of the individual, or the person learns to be self-directing in daily self-care (Caley et al, 1980).

KEY ELEMENTS OF THE PLAN

The nursing plan provides both direction and guidance for the patient and nurse, and identifies appropriate personnel to be assigned the prescribed activities. It is the vehicle through which the balance between self-care ability and self-care demand can be restored. Egan (1985) describes three stages of the helping process – exploring, understanding and acting – through which the patient and helper pass.

The type and extent of nursing intervention varies between patients. The nurse should therefore negotiate with the patient and family to determine the most effective method of meeting the patient's self-care demands.

Consideration is given to the nature of the self-care deficit and the ability of the patient to re-establish self-care. As mentioned in Chapter 3, a deficit in self-care ability arises when the patient lacks the necessary knowledge, skill or motivation to meet self-care demands.

The emphasis of a holistic and patient-centred approach is self-evident in this model.

TYPE OF NURSING INTERVENTION

Orem (1985) described three systems of nursing, reflecting different levels of self-care ability. The first system is referred to as *wholly compensatory* and applies to patients who are able to carry out little or no self-care. An unconscious or seriously ill person would fall into this category.

A *partly compensatory* system of care requires both nurse and patient to be involved. The patient's family or friends should also play an active role. Nursing is geared to maximizing what the patient can perform in the way of self-care, while compensating for self-care deficits. The nursing care will therefore change as the patient's health status and self-care ability alter.

The third system of intervention is the *educative supportive* nursing role. Intervention provides a framework by means of which the patient can acquire or develop the necessary skill, knowledge and motivation to achieve an optimum level of self-care. This system involves little 'hands on' care; it is mostly a teaching function.

The plan of care for Mr Charles (see Chapter 3) combined the partly compensatory and educative supportive systems. Mr Charles was able to maintain a certain level of self-care, but required assistance with some of his universal self-care (see p. 40) and needed additional knowledge and skill to re-establish self-care, and restore his self-esteem and dignity. Throughout his period of hospitalization Mr Charles assumed a major role in meeting his self-care demands. In practice, I have found that the majority of patients, when given the opportunity to retain control over their care, do so enthusiastically and usually require only minimal assistance to achieve optimum self-care.

PROVIDING ASSISTANCE

The nurse plans care with the patient in a variety of ways, aiming to assist patients who are incontinent either to maintain or to re-establish their balance between self-care demand and self-care ability. The level and type of involvement will vary as the patient progresses from incontinence to continence or learns to contain their incontinence, thereby establishing their self-care ability.

This is achieved by:

1 Doing or acting for the individual.
2 Providing direction or guidance.
3 Giving physical and psychological support.
4 Creating an environment conducive to self-care and development.
5 Teaching or counselling the individual.

RESOURCES

People are a most important resource. Individual strengths and weaknesses need to be established and the family's co-operation sought when helping to meet the self-care deficits. However, incontinence frequently causes severe tension and conflict within the family unit and it is not uncommon for the incontinent member of the family to be deeply resented for his or her disability. It is therefore ironic that members of the family are often expected by health care professionals to meet many of the patient's nursing needs, without any thought being given to their ability to provide the necessary care or their willingness to accept the role of informal carer.

During the planning phase, it is essential for the successful outcome of the plan that the nurse should understand the relationships between individual family members and their attitudes to the patient. Furthermore the nurse must not only be acceptable to the patient and family but must also have their permission to play an active and effective role within the host unit. Bridger (1981), recognized the importance of this in developing relationships with others.

CO-ORDINATING FUNCTION

The nurse is usually the person who undertakes the role of care co-ordinator. Ideally this should be on a basis of consultation and negotiation between the patient and others who are requested to be involved in the provision of care. All members of the team should have a clear understanding of what is required of them, why it is required, how their intervention fits in and complements that of others and how the level of success will be evaluated. The quality of the care plan can be enhanced by adopting a system of goal planning.

GOAL PLANNING

Goals are referred to in a variety of ways, and may mean different things to different people. Nurses often use terms like nursing aims, objectives, expected outcomes, whereas patients may refer to goals as things they hope will happen. A simple definition of a goal is an aim or end toward which activity is directed. Human action is characterized by individuals striving towards the attainment of their goals in both health and illness.

The type of goals set in the self-care model are patient-centred and developed through negotiation between patient, family – with his or her consent – and nurse. The relationship between the therapeutic outcome and patient involvement in goal setting is described by Willer et al (1976). It should be remembered that not everyone will be willing to be involved in goal planning and setting, and may not even understand the concept. One way of involving the appropriate people and facilitating understanding and co-operation is to ask those who wish to be involved how they perceive the situation and what they think could be done about it. The nurse should then assess the level of understanding and clarify areas of uncertainty.

When goals are formulated it is important for the nurse to remember that they must be patient-centred – they are goals for the *patient* to achieve. What the *nurse* will do is a nursing intervention and is carried out to assist the patient achieve the self-care goal.

People who are incontinent may have a wide range of problems associated with a deficit of their self-care ability. The nurse, after negotiation with the patient, is likely to draw up a care plan with an equally broad range of goals. The following criteria for goal setting are similar to those advocated by other authors, such as Egan (1985).

Criteria for the formulation of goals

A goal should include:

1 A clear and concise statement about a proposed action.
2 A means to measure or verify the outcome. (Individuals should always be able to tell if they have attained their goal.)
3 Lines of action that are realistic and achievable.
4 A clearly specified time limit for attainment.
5 Actions that do not violate the individual's personal values or cultural beliefs.
6 The means of promoting self-esteem by making the individual feel more adequate in some way on attainment of the goal.

Goal attainment

The level of frustration experienced by many incontinent people who are striving to attain the ultimate goal of re-establishing continence can be reduced by breaking down main goals into small sequential steps, each one within the individual's reach.

For example, Mrs Black (Fig. 4.1) had urgency and at times urge incontinence. One of the main goals that had been set and agreed between herself and the nurse was to re-establish a more normal voiding pattern. This was to be achieved by using bladder retraining techniques (discussed in Chapter 5) and required the patient to void at set times during the day. During the early part of the retraining programme Mrs Black, like many others who use this technique, found herself unable at times to 'hold on' until the set time and experienced episodes of incontinence. However, her disappointment and frustration were minimized because the set interval periods for voiding were based on information obtained from her

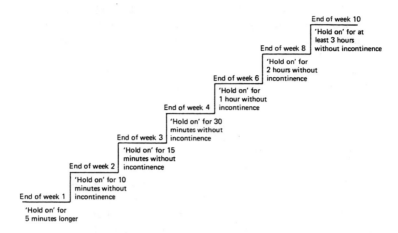

Fig. 4.1. *Steps taken by Mrs Black to achieve a more normal voiding pattern.*

continence chart and were sufficiently frequent to enable her to achieve success within the specified period.

Mrs Black was able to monitor her own progress by keeping and referring to her continence charts and this helped sustain her motivation.

Timing

The need to have a clearly specified time for goal attainment was mentioned earlier. Some goals are achieved within a day or two; others over weeks or even months.

For example, Mr David (Fig. 4.2) had moderate incontinence. After an initial assessment it was agreed that the symptom could be managed by wearing a penile sheath as a short-term intervention until a thorough investigation could be completed and the results analysed.

Short-term goals which meet the criteria given on page 79 offer immediate hope and reassurance to the patient and family that something can be and is being done to improve the situation. This helps to reduce the despair and frustration that so frequently accompany bladder or bowel dysfunction.

Goals also have the advantage that they offer clarification of what may be a confusing situation. Achievement of short-

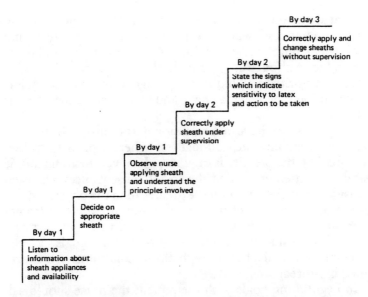

Fig. 4.2. *Steps taken by Mr David to correct his knowledge and skill deficit in order to re-establish self-care ability.*

term goals helps to sustain motivation, encourages a positive attitude to continence promotion or the management of incontinence and can help evaluate the success of the planned intervention.

It is, however, important that the patient specifies with the help and support of the nurse what his or her *long-term* goals are as this will identify a framework within which the patient and nurse can function. Long-term goals also help to determine what future resources might be required, giving those concerned sufficient time to make the necessary preparations.

Determining goal priorities

One of the problems which faces both the nurse and patient is deciding which goals are most important and therefore need to be met first. (Useful guidelines are provided by Maslow, 1954 and Redman, 1975.) In practice – from my own experience – this is often far more difficult than it may appear, and may require the nurse to support, guide and advise the patient if the goals are to be achieved. I have known many patients and nurses who attempt to alleviate all the presenting problems simultaneously, with the sad result that failure is inevitable. Although it is difficult, the plan of care must give order of priority to all of the wide range of complex problems an incontinent person may have and try and solve them one at a time.

As nurses we have a professional responsibility to help patients overcome such difficulties. Where a problem is life-threatening, the priority is obvious. However, incontinence is rarely life-threatening and the social consequences are often considered by the patient to be greater than the physical ones. Many of the models of nursing currently used have a framework for the assessment of patient needs; this could act as a crude but systematic means of prioritizing goals, as the assessment usually begins with those conditions which are most life-threatening.

In negotiating goals with the patient the nurse should ask what the patient sees as first priority. The chances are that this may be very different from the nurse's perception of priorities; this requires careful negotiation before a mutually agreeable set of priorities can be arrived at. As goals are achieved, the re-assessment and re-ordering of priorities are necessary to ensure that the overall goal is still attainable, and that the patient retains responsibility and control for his or her own care programme. This fact is implicit in the model of self-care detailed by Orem, and is essential in the promotion of continence and for the effective management of incontinence.

Conflicting goals

The involvement of other health care professionals and the patient's family has already been mentioned, together with the co-ordinating role of the nurse. Unless co-operation is obtained from all those involved and a joint consultative decision is made about priorities, there is a danger that conflicting goals will be set. This may result in the patient not progressing favourably towards the attainment of continence. If the incontinent person appears reluctant to agree priorities, it is important that he or she is not labelled as difficult or uncooperative. The nurse should always seek to find answers as to why the patient feels reluctant. Does the individual, for example, feel unable to cope with what is being asked? Does he or she lack the knowledge or skill needed to meet the goal requirements? Do the requirements violate the patient's personal values or beliefs? It may be that the method indicated for achievement is unacceptable, rather than its priority or end-results. Carers must not impose their view of what is right on the patient; goals must at all times remain patient-centred and be stated in terms of patient actions.

THE WRITTEN PLAN

The variety of formats for care plans is quite extensive and usually complements the underlying philosophy of care. However, it is not the size, shape, format or where the plan is kept that offers the key to successful patient care, but rather its content and clarity. Ideally, there is one plan of care which should depict the intervention of all the different disciplines involved. Unfortunately despite their often close working relationship, the majority of disciplines prefer to keep separate plans of care, which can make communication and co-ordination more difficult for the patient and nurse. Despite the diversity of format, many outline plans contain similar components:

1 Date when the intervention was prescribed and name of prescriber.
2 What the intervention consists of, described in sequential steps.
3 Who is to carry out the prescribed action – patient, nurse, relatives, physiotherapist, doctor, occupational therapist, social worker.
4 Where the activity is to be performed.
5 When it is to take place.
6 How the patient and appropriate carer will know when the action has been successful.
7 Date when the intervention is to be reassessed or discontinued and the name of the person evaluating the outcome.

In other words, the care plan clearly and concisely identifies the criteria for intervention, the conditions under which the action or behaviour is to take place and the method of evaluating the outcome.

SUMMARY

The condition that validates the existence of a requirement for nursing (Orem, 1980) is the absence of ability to maintain a balance between self-care ability and self-care demand.

This chapter has attempted to apply a systematic approach to the design and plan of nursing intervention in order to bring about a favourable change in the health status of an individual with incontinence who may have a wide range of self-care deficits. The underlying assumption is that self-care must be based on knowledge rather than whim; patients must be able to make informed decisions about their care (Campbell, 1984).

References

Bridger H. (1981). Consultative work with communication and organizations. In *Management and Managing – A Dynamic Approach*. Walton M. (ed.). London: Harper Row.

Caley J. M., Dirkson M., Engalla M. et al (1980). The Orem self care nursing model. In *Conceptual Models for Nursing Practice*. (Riehl J. P., Callista R., eds). London: Appleton Century Crofts.

Campbell C. (1984). Orem's story. *Nursing Mirror*, 159, 13, 28–30.

Egan G. (1985). *The Skilled Helper* 3rd edn. Monterey, California: Brooks/Cole.

Maslow A. (1954). *Motivation and Personality*. New York: Harper & Row.

Orem D. (1980). *Nursing: Concepts of Practice*. New York: McGraw Hill.

Orem D. (1985). *Nursing: Concepts of Practice* 3rd edn. New York: McGraw Hill.

Redman B. K. (1975). Guidelines for quality of care in patient education. *Canadian Nurse*, 71, 19–21.

Willer B., Miller G. H. (1976). Client involvement in goal setting and its relationship to therapeutic outcome. *Journal of Clinical Psychology*, 32, (3), 687–90.

Bibliography

Aggleton P., Chalmers H. (1985). Models and theories 5. Orem's self care model. *Nursing Times*, January 2nd, 81, (1), 36–9.

Knowles S. M. (1980). *Modern Practice of Adult Education from Pedagogy to Andragogy* (revised edn). Cambridge: Adult Education Company.

Little D. E., Carnevali D. L. (1976). *Nursing Care Planning.* Philadelphia: J. B. Lippincott.

Revill S., Blunden R. (1980). *Goal Planning with Mentally Handicapped People in the Community. Report on an Evaluation of the Uses of Goal Planning Technique by Health Visitors. Report 9. Mental Handicap in Wales.* Wales: Applied Research Unit.

Tschudin V. (1982). *Counselling Skills for Nurses.* London: Bailliere Tindall.

5

Intervention to promote continence

The implementation of a planned intervention is the fourth stage in the nursing process. The aim of this chapter is to provide guidelines and advice on a range of treatments and interventions (excluding catheterization, which is discussed in Chapter 6) to assist the patient to regain continence and re-establish the balance between self-care demand and self-care ability. Teaching methods to promote and maintain self and family help are discussed in Chapter 7.

Two themes which run concurrently throughout this text are the patient-centred and multidisciplinary approach in the promotion and maintenance of self-care.

Sufficient accurate information should have been obtained about the patient from the history examination and assessment details to enable determination of the type of intervention. As discussed in Chapter 4, intervention can be wholly or partly compensatory or educative supportive. The type and areas of intervention discussed in this text include:

1 Assisting the patient to eliminate in the appropriate place and receptacle.
2 Advising the patient on how to achieve a balanced diet and correct fluid intake.
3 Teaching the patient how to avoid urinary tract infection.
4 Supporting and assisting the patient to re-establish a normal pattern of faecal and urinary elimination.
5 Counselling and supporting the patient and family to

overcome emotional factors which may inhibit continence promotion.

6 Acting on behalf of the patient to correct iatrogenic factors.
7 Teaching, advising and supporting the patient on techniques to promote continence.

A change of environment or normal routine can affect the ability of an individual to promote or maintain self-care ability. This is often apparent when patients are admitted to hospital if they are not involved in the plan of care or encouraged to maintain self-care. This effect should be borne in mind when caring for newly hospitalized patients, especially if they are elderly.

THE TOILET

The majority of homes in the UK have an indoor toilet. However, not everyone finds it convenient or easy to get to or use the facility. Even greater problems can arise when people are required to use communal toilets, especially where there is a lack of privacy. This in itself can often be a common cause of incontinence; patient care should start by ensuring this simple detail has been carefully considered.

It is useful to have the occupational therapist and physiotherapist assess the patient with the nurse as both may be involved in assisting the patient. If, for example, the patient has difficulty in rising from a chair or getting out of bed, then the technique used to carry out this action should be observed. Often simple advice on how to improve present technique is all that may be required. If the height of the chair is unsuitable, then advice on seating can be given to enable the patient to select a chair that will overcome the problem. A rope ladder attached to the end of the bed can be especially helpful in assisting some patients who have difficulty getting into a sitting or upright position.

Occasionally a patient may require some form of mechanical assistance in order to be able to get up from a chair. A number of such chairs are available. The mechanism for operating the chair seat is usually located on the arm, and once activated seat and patient are gently manoeuvred upwards and forwards, so enabling the patient to stand up. As many patients who require the use of such aids also have difficulty in maintaining their balance, a walking frame will probably be required. Walking aids come in a variety of shapes and sizes and if selected and used properly can greatly increase the patient's confidence and mobility. A few seconds difference in getting to the toilet can result in the patient either remaining continent or becoming incontinent.

Having established ways to enable the patient to stand and maintain balance, the next potential deficits of self-care are associated with obstacles that may be encountered along the way, and the inability to walk unaided to the toilet.

Obstructions can be common and in situations when seconds count, a puddle on the floor or a soiled garment is often the result of delay. Obstacles are not put there deliberately to hinder the person and often all that is required is for the nurse or therapist to explain the problem and they can be readily removed. In my experience most people are usually only too pleased to assist if it helps promote continence. However objects do not usually get moved unless attention is drawn to them as a potential cause of incontinence.

Many elderly people experience difficulty in walking for a variety of medical reasons. However, it is not uncommon to find a high proportion of people compounding mobility problems by wearing inappropriate footwear, such as ill-fitting shoes or slippers which interfere with walking. Advice should always be offered. It is perhaps unnecessary to mention that the nurse or therapist should be cautious when discussing alternative types of footwear as the price range of shoes is extensive and some fall far outside the income of many people.

Feet are possibly the most neglected part of the body and can seriously impair mobility unless properly cared for. Long or ingrowing toe nails, callouses and the like can be very painful and the nurse or therapist may advise the patient to seek help from a chiropodist if appropriate (Judd, 1989).

The next potential self-care deficit relates to the removal of appropriate clothing and the act of sitting down on the toilet seat. The undoing of zips, buttons or other types of fasteners requires the patient to have skilful flexion and rotation of the hands. Unfortunately many people lose the fine degree of dexterity required to perform this function and although they may get to the toilet without voiding along the way, the time spent in undoing garments and removing articles of clothing often takes longer than the patient can 'hold on'. The use of Velcro as an alternative to other types of fasteners usually proves very successful and is relatively cheap and easy to fit. Sometimes women require advice on the suitability of clothing or on techniques for quickly removing outer and undergarments.

The height and type of toilet seat should have been assessed for suitability. A person may, for example, have painful knee or hip joints and find bending difficult. In this situation the use of a raised seat may be beneficial. The occupational therapist would probably be the most appropriate person to advise the patient on what would be most suitable.

If the seat is too high, then a footstool could be used to enable the patient to sit in the appropriate upright position with feet supported. Some patients, particularly elderly people, lose confidence and become frightened when going to sit down on the seat, and tend to grab at objects such as another person, toilet roll holder or door handle, losing their balance as a result. Much can be done to prevent this situation by increasing the patient's confidence, and by the use of grip rails to assist the patient in lowering him- or herself on to the seat, or to give leverage when standing up again.

In some situations it may be advisable to suggest the use of either a mechanical or electrically operated toilet seat which will manoeuvre the patient upwards and forwards. The Looabililty (Fig. 5.1; Warren Hooker, Poole) is strongly moulded in hygienic thermoformed plastic and designed to replace an ordinary toilet seat. It has a simple operating lever so that the seat can be left unlocked in the upright position, ready to ease the patient gently down; alternatively it can be left locked down, resembling an ordinary toilet seat. Operating the seat to stand up is extremely easy; the patient unlocks the side lever, places the feet firmly on the floor, leaning forward slightly. The spring-powered seat provides the exact help required to stand upright.

Toilet paper

This almost seems too elementary to mention, but it is surprising how many patients have soiled undergarments

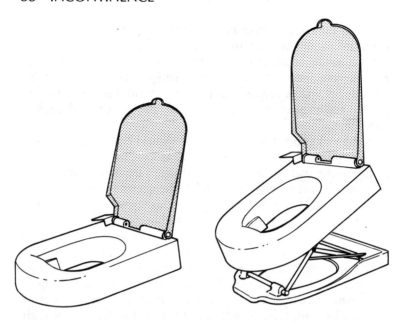

Fig. 5.1. *The Warren Hooker Looability.* **A** Locked down; **B** Unlocked up position. The seat is spring-powered.

because of absent or inadequate toilet paper, or if the individual lacks the dexterity necessary to reach the paper and use it properly. Many patients find the position of the toilet roll holder not easily accessible, and often have to perform precarious movements to grasp and tear off some paper. Some patients experience difficulty in wiping themselves (this problem is discussed in more detail in Chapter 9). It may be helpful to the patient if the toilet roll holder is moved to a more suitable position and individual tissues are used, as opposed to a roll. The extent to which these minor adjustments are carried out depends very much on where the individual lives – own home, rest or nursing home or hospital – and the commitment and insight of those involved.

If a person is unable to get to the toilet then there is a range of alternative receptacles which can be used; these are discussed in Chapter 9.

DIET AND FLUIDS

Some people can be helped to regain continence by making alterations in their eating and drinking habits. Problems occur if the individual drinks either too much or too little fluid. The latter often happens if the person lacks motivation and cannot be bothered to make or get a drink; others may be unable to undertake this activity due to physical or mental impairment. Of significance in promoting continence are those patients who deliberately restrict fluid intake to treat the incontinence. Apart from dehydration the lack of fluid is more likely to aggravate the bladder problem, especially if the urine is concentrated and irritates the bladder mucosa. If the individual is unable to get or make drinks then flasks or bottles of fluid can be prepared and left near to hand by carers. The importance of fluid intake must be carefully discussed with the patient.

On the other hand many elderly people drink copious amounts of fluids throughout the day, some of which (tea or coffee) act as stimulants, increasing the chances of incontinence, especially if the person has problems of mobility. The patient's fluid intake should be calculated for a 24-hour period as it is important to know what and how much was drunk and when. Most patients are happy to co-operate and keep a record of their drinking habit for a few days. Advice can then be given to correct any imbalance; patients who have a high fluid intake and suffer from nocturia might be advised to reduce fluids after 6 or 7 p.m. to possibly one cup of beverage. Some nurses suggest that the patient should have no fluids after 5 or 6 p.m., which is extreme and often distressing to the patient. The patient who suffers from nocturia should always be advised to empty the bladder immediately before going to sleep.

Diet plays an equally important role in the promotion of continence. The nurse should know the patient's normal dietary pattern and assess the patient for evidence of oral or dental problems such as tooth decay, mouth ulcers, ill-fitting dentures and the like, which may inhibit the individual from taking a balanced diet. If necessary the patient should be advised to see a dentist.

A dietician may be involved in helping the patient plan a

balanced diet. Fibre is essential to promote regular bowel function. However, patients will need considerable teaching and encouragement if they are to realize the advantages of changing diet. Flatulence problems in particular need tactful explanation to reduce the risk of the patient returning to previous dietary habits.

Specific problems that may arise for elderly or disabled people and children are discussed in Chapter 9.

Insufficient intake of fluids and the appropriate foods can give rise to constipation which, as mentioned in Chapter 2, is a precipitating factor in incontinence.

CONSTIPATION

Constipation, if left untreated, can result in the individual developing faecal impaction and episodes of spurious diarrhoea. Many people appear quite obsessed about regular bowel actions and frequently resort to taking a variety of medicines to keep themselves regular. Unfortunately the overuse of laxatives often gives rise to loss of normal function.

The causes and effects of faecal incontinence have been discussed in Chapter 2 and the importance of an accurate history, assessment and examination in Chapter 3. Intervention should be structured towards the patient goal of re-establishing a more normal pattern of elimination and should include an educational and supportive input, so that once a normal pattern has been established it may be maintained. If the patient has a self-care deficit its cause must be discovered first. In Chapter 3 Mr Charles presented with what he thought was diarrhoea; in fact he had faecal impaction with spurious diarrhoea. A rectal examination revealed large quantities of hard faecal matter. As the rectum had been distended for quite a while this had caused the internal and external anal sphincters to become inhibited and therefore relaxed, allowing faecal fluid to leak out. This leakage is known as spurious diarrhoea, and is due to hard faecal matter irritating the bowel, causing the excessive production of mucus which then combines with the bacterial flora in the gut to produce a foul-smelling fluid. Not all patients with constipation have a distended rectum; if the patient has faecal overflow this can give rise to incorrect treatment for diarrhoea, thus worsening the situation. If diagnosis is uncertain, then a straight x-ray of the abdomen will show up faecal impaction.

What nursing intervention should be taken to assist Mr Charles to regain a more normal pattern of defecation? Before continuing with Mr Charles's case history, simple remedies to treat and prevent constipation will be discussed. The importance of an adequate fluid intake and a well balanced diet with sufficient roughage has already been mentioned. Most cases of simple constipation can be treated by increasing the intake of dietary fibre. Unprocessed wheat bran sprinkled or mixed in food and taken with a sufficient quantity of fluids will give bulk to the stools, leading to an increase in peristaltic action within the gut. The nurse or dietician must stress the need for adequate fluid intake, otherwise intestinal obstruction may arise. The patient may prefer to eat bran, or the high fibre bread, biscuits or cakes that are now available. Providing the patient's general state of health permits, a gradual and gentle increase in exercise will improve bowel activity and reduce the transit time of food through the bowel. The advice of a physiotherapist about exercise is often very useful to the patient, and can provide the necessary motivation.

The need for a correct height toilet seat or the use of a footstool to aid positioning and defecation have been already discussed. Privacy has been mentioned but requires elaboration. Children at school find privacy in the toilet extremely difficult, if not impossible to achieve, which may lead to problems at an early age. Many withhold defecation until they return home, rather than risk ridicule or teasing in the toilet. School toilets often have only partly partitioned walls which allow children to peep under or over the top and doors do not always close proberly. Advice from the health visitor and school nurse to the local education authority could help bring about improvement.

In ward situations nurses remember to draw curtains around the patient but frequently forget that this visual barrier does not provide a barrier for noise or odour, which are possibly the two elements of elimination that cause the greatest distress and embarrassment to patients. Similar problems can arise from living in a communal dwelling. Whenever possible the patient should be helped to get to the toilet, rather than made to use commodes or bedpans in the ward area. Wright (1974) found that patients who had to use these types of receptacles were far more anxious and concerned than those who were able to eliminate in the toilet.

The general state of cleanliness of the toilet can inhibit defecation, especially if the seats are soiled or broken, the pan is dirty, toilet paper is absent and the air is foul-smelling. Broken windows and door locks can make the individual feel a lack of privacy. In theory this type of situation is easy to remedy; in practice it becomes far more difficult as it requires the constant commitment of those providing and using the facilities to keep them properly maintained.

If the patient at home is unable to keep the toilet and general living quarters clean and no other assistance is available, the occupational therapist may be able to advise on domestic gadgets to help perform general cleaning activities, or the assistance of a home help may be required.

If the patient has haemorrhoids or any other anorectal condition which may cause pain during elimination, advice should be given that medical help and treatment should be sought. Withholding elimination may occur due to the pain involved and will therefore lead to constipation.

Laxatives are often misused by both patients and professional carers (Table 5.1). Care should be given to the selection of laxatives; it should be determined by the nature of the patient's constipation. If we consider the case of Mr Charles (see Chapter 3), he had a microlette enema every morning for 6 days until the impaction was completely dislodged and the faecal matter eliminated. In practice, both micro and phosphate small enemas give good results. However, I find many nurses only give one or two of the micro phosphate enemas and then consider the bowel to be emptied as the results are usually 'good'; however, it is important to ensure that the bowel is completely clear. This can usually be established by a straight abdominal x-ray.

Soap and water enemas should be avoided as they can cause inflammation of the mucous membrane. The need for a nurse or anyone to perform a manual removal of faeces from a patient should be rare as the correct use of laxatives should avoid this unpleasant, degrading and distressing procedure.

The use of bulk-forming agents should only commence

Table 5.1.   Categories and examples of commonly used laxatives

Category	Example
Hydrophilic or bulk-forming agents	Natural bran, Isogel, Fybogel, methylcellulose
Chemical stimulants or irritants	Bisacodyl, senna, Dorbanex, Normax
Lubricants or softening agents	Dioctyl, castor oil
Fluid-retaining or osmotic	Lactulose, Duphalac, Petrolagar
Miscellaneous	
Administration rectally	Suppositories
Lucricant and softening agents	Glycerol
Stimulants	Bisacodyl, Dulcolax
Enemas	
Lubricant and softening agent	Fletchers – various types
Osmotic action	Micro – various types

when the bowl has been cleared, otherwise the increased stool formation can exacerbate the impaction. Patients should also be advised that these agents usually take between 2 and 3 days after ingestion to become effective.

The nurse should discuss with the patient ways to help establish a normal pattern of elimination. This is especially important if the individual has diminished rectal sensation or tends to ignore and suppress the desire to defecate.

Senna and cascara have long been found in family medicine cupboards; both are laxatives which act as chemical irritants on the bowel mucosa to stimulate and increase mobility. The intensity of the action frequently causes quite severe abdominal cramps. The urine is often coloured red when these preparations are taken. Their prolonged use should be discouraged as they may cause loss of normal gut motility. There are a number of alternative drugs that have less dramatic effects, although prolonged use of any irritant laxative is not to be encouraged due to its harmful effect over a period of time on the mucosa of the gut.

Liquid paraffin and castor oil are both faecal softeners and have been in use for many years. However, the harmful side-effects of liquid paraffin are well documented and include binding of fat-soluble vitamins so that they are not absorbed and faecal incontinence. Liquid paraffin should not be used by professional carers. Nurses are advised to enquire whether the patient uses this laxative, and offer appropriate advice if the answer is yes. Castor oil is also not recommended for use on a regular basis, as it can produce excessive peristaltic activity and a complete clearance of the large bowel. It is, however, often used as a preoperative preparation for patients undergoing bowel surgery.

SELF-RESPECT

Incontinence can quickly destroy an individual's confidence and self-respect. An important and essential aspect of intervention is to assist the patient to regain confidence and self-respect, without which normalcy is unattainable.

There are many strategies a nurse can use, and these are well documented in the literature as indicated in previous chapters. The first step in the helping process is to gain the patient's acceptance and trust. This may take some time to achieve and requires tact and patience on the part of the nurse. One important point for the nurse to remember is never to get so involved in a conversation that overall control of the situation is lost.

Always listen carefully to what the patient is saying. It may be helpful to paraphrase back to the patient what you think he or she said to you. This is useful in clarifying your own understanding of what has been said and in getting the patient to consider whether what you have said is what they intended to say.

Never be tempted to interrupt patients, especially if they begin to say things like 'I smell', 'I can't go on like this any longer'. Nurses often want to show they care and tend to interrupt this type of conversation by saying things like: 'No, you don't smell' or 'You'll be all right, I'll help you'. It is much better to let patients say all the things that they want to express, whilst you quietly sit there looking attentive. The reasons behind the patient's thinking should be gently explored. Once you have achieved this type of relationship, you will be better able to encourage, support and if need be, offer guidance and advice to help the patient regain self-confidence and respect.

Remember that the nurse can also become the object of the patient's anger and frustration. If this situation arises, the nurse should follow the advice given above and resist the temptation to interrupt the patient, who should be allowed to ventilate anger or frustration. Only then can a constructive dialogue begin.

URINARY TRACT INFECTION

Most urinary tract infections involve pathogenic organisms ascending via the urethra to the bladder and possibly via the ureters to the kidneys. The most common invading organisms and presenting clinical symptoms were discussed in Chapter 2. Urinary infection following catheterization is discussed in Chapter 6. Intervention should aim to eradicate the infection and advise the patient how to treat the presenting symptoms and prevent their recurrence.

A mid-stream specimen of urine should be obtained and sent for culture and organism sensitivity to the pathology department. Many doctors prefer to wait for the pathology department report which indicates the type and number of organisms before deciding on the appropriate medication. Drugs frequently prescribed include co-trimoxazole, natidixic acid, nitrofurantoin and ampicillin. It is important that the patient understands when the drug is to be taken, for example, many antibiotics like nitrofurantoin should be given with or immediately after a meal as they can cause irritation of the alimentrary tract and gastric upsets. Most patients with a urinary tract infection should be encouraged to drink between 3 and 5 litres of fluid a day, which can be difficult if they feel lethargic and nauseous.

Should the patient have difficulty washing and wiping the perineal area, the use of toilet aids can be helpful. In most instances simple advice on hand-washing and general points of hygiene are usually sufficient. Unfortunately, it is not only the patient or relations who require education on hand-washing. A study by Wright (1974) found that over one-third of hospital patients confined to bed received no offer of hand-washing facilities following elimination.

PELVIC FLOOR EXERCISES

Many female patients with mild or moderate stress incontinence can be helped to regain continence by correctly exercising the muscles of the pelvic floor. The muscles of the pelvic floor and perineum are constantly active in helping to support the pelvic organs and increase intra-abdominal pressure. The muscular structure of the pelvis is often described as hammock-shaped, formed by the levator ani muscles, urogenital diaphragm and superficial muscles (Fig. 5.2 and 5.3). The most important muscles when exercising the pelvic floor are the group collectively referred to as the levator ani (pubococcygeus, iliococcygeus and ischiococcygeus). For a variety of reasons (childbirth, straining at stool, hormonal changes,

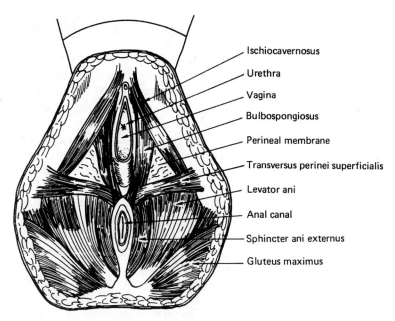

Fig. 5.2. *Musculature of the perineum – female.*

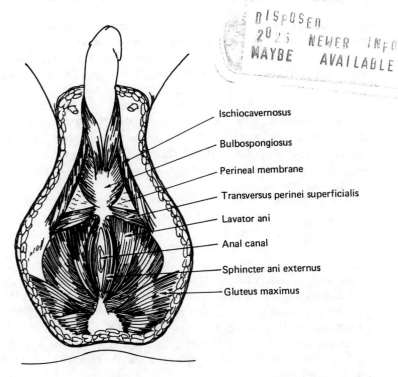

Ischiocavernosus

Bulbospongiosus

Perineal membrane

Transversus perinei superficialis

Lavator ani

Anal canal

Sphincter ani externus

Gluteus maximus

Fig. 5.3. *Musculature of the perineum – male.*

surgical trauma) the muscles lose their tone, become lax and sag.

The patient should have the pelvic floor described to her with the aid of simple diagram or cupping of hands and the benefit of pelvic floor exercises should be explained. A useful book for patient education is *Regaining Bladder Control*, written by Montgomery (1983). It is important that the patient understands she will have a major part to play in achieving success, and has the necessary motivation to continue with the exercises at regular intervals each day for several months. Once the patient decides she wants to try this therapy the nurse or physiotherapist must obtain her permission before performing a vaginal examination.

The patient should lie in a supine position with legs apart and knees drawn upwards. The perineum and vagina should be checked for signs of inflammation or irritation together with leakage and bulging at the introitus on coughing or pushing. If the patient has a cystocele or rectocele (prolapse of the anterior or posterior vaginal wall) or urethrocele, this is confirmed by digital examination of the vagina. A severe prolapse can affect the chances of successful attainment of continence; however, if the patient is aware that she may not regain continence but remains motivated to try, then she should be encouraged to do so. If surgery is required the exercises will help the patient during the postoperative recovery phase as the blood flow and muscle tone in that area will be improved.

The strength of the levator ani muscles is assessed by placing two fingers in the introitus. The patient is then asked to stop the examiner from pulling out the fingers. Many women find it difficult to exert more than a momentary twitch; others can produce a firm squeeze. Sometimes it is easier for the patient to imagine she has diarrhoea in order to help her locate the right muscles. Once the patient can identify the correct muscles and feels the sensation of the pelvic floor rising upwards and backwards towards the spine she can commence the exercises. It may take some time for the patient to feel this, and she may require a lot of reassurance and encouragement.

Some professional carers use an instrument called a perimeter (Shepherd and Montgomery, 1983) instead of digital assessment to determine the strength of the muscles as it provides a visual recording which the patient may also find helpful. A perimeter is a compressible rubber air chamber approximately 20 cm long which is connected to a manometer by a rubber tube. The base of the chamber fits against the perineum.

Another exercise to isolate the pelvic floor muscles involves asking the patient to interrupt micturition mid-stream. This action helps to exercise the pelvic muscles, as well as identify the sensation that accompanies pelvic floor contraction. This exercise is performed in the toilet. When the patient is seated comfortably with her legs astride, she stops the flow mid-stream for a few seconds then recommences. Many patients with pelvic floor weakness may not immediately be able to stop the flow. However, with practice this is attainable.

Success will depend on the patient establishing and maintaining a regular exercise programme. The pelvic floor contraction exercises can be carried out whilst the woman is standing, sitting or lying with the legs slightly astride. The patient is instructed how to close her vagina and anal passage by firmly contracting the pelvic floor muscles. This position is held for the count of 5, then relaxed. This exercise is repeated 4–5 times each hour throughout the day. The patient should notice an improvement within 3 months; most women with mild to moderate stress incontinence are continent within 12 months.

Pelvic floor exercises can also be of value to male patients with post-prostatectomy incontinence. Physiotherapists have a major role to play in teaching pelvic floor exercises (Harrison, 1983).

ELECTROTHERAPY TECHNIQUES

Electrotheraphy techniques are sometimes used in conjunction with pelvic floor exercises to promote continence. However, research is still in its infancy, and hence there is a dearth of available literature. The work of Shepherd (1980) highlights evidence of its successful use, although many professional carers remain sceptical as to its value. Faradism involves the use of a vaginal electrode probe which produces a low frequency current to initiate a pelvic floor contraction.

Interferential therapy is thought to stimulate the autonomic and pudendal nerves supplying the neuromuscular tissues in the deep pelvic floor and urethra. Unlike faradism, this technique is non-invasive (McGuire, 1975).

BLADDER AND TOILET TRAINING PROGRAMMES

The ultimate aim of any bladder or toilet training programme is to help the patient re-establish the goal of continence or at least to contain incontinence. The success of such programmes depends on them being designed to meet the individual needs of the patient.

Unfortunately the profession appears to have a major task in trying to educate its members on the appropriate use of available techniques. Many institutions, particularly those caring for elderly or handicapped people, adopt one regime and apply it to all patients, regardless of their individual problems.

A record should be kept over a number of days to determine the patient's voiding pattern. The patient's history and assessment should indicate mental alterness as well as problems such as underlying bladder dysfunction, constipation or urinary tract infection. If present, these problems must be tackled before the method of toilet training and its implications can be discussed and agreement reached between the patient and nurse.

Set or variable interval toileting

This type of regime is useful for patients who forget at times to go to the toilet, or who suffer from urgency or urge incontinence. The times when the patient is to void are clearly indicated on the continence chart, and should be designed to meet the individual's requirements. For example, if the patient is usually wet at 7.30 a.m. then voiding should be tried at 7 a.m. Setting toilet times before the recorded episodes of incontinence on the assessment charts is important to the success of set interval toileting. It may be that an individual has more episodes of incontinence in the morning than the afternoon. Therefore, the interval between toileting can be longer in the afternoon. As continence is achieved it is important to extend the intervals until an optimum interval of between 3 and 4 hours has been achieved without incontinent episodes. This may take several months to achieve, during which time the patient may have many setbacks and require considerable support from family and carers.

Some medical and nursing staff consider it helpful to commence the programme with the patient in hospital (Frewin, 1978; Jarvis and Millar, 1980). It is important to monitor the patient's progress carefully and adjust the programme in the light of the available information.

An alternative programme is to ask the patient to extend the period between the first sensation of wanting to void and the act of voiding. Mrs Black (see p. 78) attained continence by using this type of programme. Patient motivation and continued commitment, even after episodes of incontinence have occurred, are the key to a successful programme and establishing continence. Without adequate support, many patients may give up and resign themselves to being incontinent.

DRUG THERAPY

Drug therapy may be used on its own or in conjunction with other forms of conservative treatment. Table 5.2 gives a range of drugs which can be used to treat various types of incontinence and urinary symptoms.

SURGICAL INTERVENTIONS

It is not within the remit of this text to discuss the range of surgical interventions which may be performed to 'cure' incontinence. However, the technique of artificial sphincter implantation (Whitehead 1984; Moore, 1985; Schreiter, 1985) now offers hope of continence to many adults and children, in particular those with spina bifida. One type of prosthesis currently available is the American Medical Systems (AMS) Sphincter 800.

The AMS Sphincter 800

The AMS Sphincter 800 urinary prosthesis consists of three parts – a cuff, a pump and a balloon (Fig. 5.4). Each part is filled with fluid and connected by silicone tubing. The cuff is either wrapped around the base of the bladder or it may be placed around the bulbous urethra in men. The pump usually lies in the scrotum of men, and in one of the labia in women. The balloon lies in the pelvic cavity near the bladder.

To operate the sphincter mechanism the patient sits or stands in the appropriate voiding position then gently squeezes the soft part of the pump several times. This action causes the fluid in the cuff to empty into the balloon. The pressure normally exerted by the cuff to the base of the bladder or bulbous urethra is now released so that urine may be voided. Once the patient stops squeezing the pump, the

Table 5.2.

Drug name	Usual dosage	Urinary symptoms to be treated	Side-effects
Propantheline (Pro-Banthine)	45–120 mg adult 15–45 mg child	Enuresis	Rarely used due to side-effects. Dry mouth, blurred vision, drowsiness, hesitancy and retention
Poldine (Nacton)	2 mg at night (child) (taken at bedtime)	Enuresis	Non-apparent
Imipramine (Tofranil)	25 mg 6–7 years; 20–25 kg. 25–50 mg 8–11 years; 25–35 kg. 50–75 mg +11 years; 35–54 kg. (taken at bedtime)	Nocturnal enuresis	Dry mouth, blurred vision, gastrointestinal upsets, as for propantheline
Flavoxate (Urispas)	200 mg t.d.s. adult Not recommended for under 12-year-olds	Dysuria Urgency Nocturia Frequency Incontinence due to inflammation or infection, cystitis, prostatitis, urethritis	Usually well tolerated. Slight nausea if taken on an empty stomach
Emepronium (Cetiprin)	200 mg t.d.s. or adult 200–400 mg nocte (3–4 week course of tablets required)	Frequency Nocturia Following trauma i.e. Radiotherapy Surgery Prostatectomy	Dry mouth, buccal ulceration, especially if tablets not taken with over 100 ml fluid

Drug name	Usual dosage	Urinary symptoms to be treated	Side-effects
Oxybutinin (Cystrin)	5 mg t.d.s. or b.d. adult 5 mg b.d. child +5	Frequency Nocturnal enuresis Unstable bladder Urgency, urge/ stress incontinence	Dry mouth, tachycardia, blurred vision, retention, constipation
Terodiline (Terolin)	12.5 mg b.d. adult Not recommended for children (continue treatment for 2–3 weeks)	Incontinence Frequency, urgency Detrusor instability Neurogenic disorders of bladder	Dry mouth, blurred vision, gastrointestinal upsets, as for propantheline
Phenoxybenzamine (Dibenyline)	10 mg b.d. adults only	Urethro-detrusor dyssynergia (failure of the urethra to open when bladder contracts causing outflow obstruction)	Severe hypotension. Patient needs careful observation
Phenylpropanolamine (Eskornade)	1 capsule b.d. adult 5 ml b.d. child 7–10 years	Stress incontinence Detrusor instability	Dry mouth
Bethanechol chloride (Myotonine)	10 mg q.d.s.	Atonic bladder	Diarrhoea Hypersalivation
Oestrogens		Senile vaginitis	

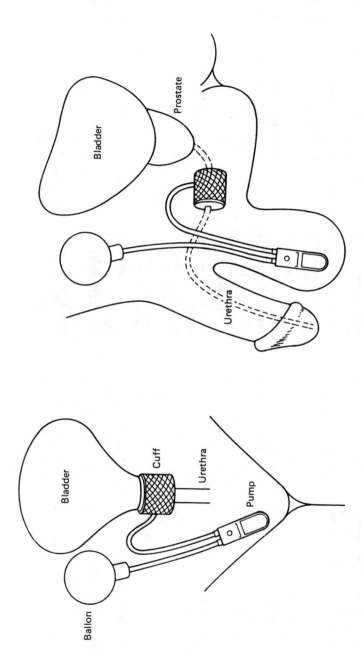

Fig. 5.4. *The American Medical Systems Sphincter 800.* **A** The cuff is implanted around the bladder neck in males and females. **B** In males, the cuff can be implanted at the bulbous urethra.

fluid will re-enter the cuff and the urine flow is inhibited. The cuff is fully inflated and continence is restored within a few moments.

SUMMARY

In this chapter I have attempted to examine some of the interventions available to regulate the incontinent patient's therapeutic self-care demands. By adopting a systematic approach to nursing care, consideration is given to the nature of the self-care deficit and ability of the patient to re-establish self-care. Thus the intervention is planned to maximize patient and family involvement and may be either of a compensatory or educative nature.

References

Frewin W. K. (1987). An objectory assessment of the unstable bladder of psychosymatic origin. *British Journal of Urology*, 50, 246–9.

Harrison F. M. (1983). Stress incontinence and the physiotherapist. *Physiotherapy*, 69, (5), 144–7.

Harrison S. (1975). Physiotherapy in the Treatment of Stress Incontinence, *Nursing Mirror*, July 10, 81, (28), 52–3.

Jarvis G. J., Millar D. R. (1980). Controlled trial of bladder drill for detrusor instability. *British Medical Journal*, 281, 1322–3.

Judd M. (1989). *Mobility: Patient Problems and Nursing Care.* Oxford: Heinemann Nursing.

McGuire W. A. (1975). Electro-therapy and exercises for stress incontinence and urinary frequency. *Physiotherapy*, 61 (10), 305–7.

Montgomery E. (1983). *Regaining Bladder Control.* Bristol: John Wright.

Moore C. (1985). Urinary incontinence and the artificial sphincter. *The Canadian Nurse*, 81, (4), 32–5.

Schreiter S. (1985). Bobath artificial sphincter. *European Urology*, 11, 294–9.

Shepherd A. M. (1980). Re-education of the muscles of the pelvic floor. In *Incontinence and its Management* (Mandelstom D. ed.) Kent: Croom Helm.

Shepherd A. M., Montgomery E. (1983). Treatment of genuine

stress incontinence with a new perimeter. *Physiotherapy*, **9** (4), 113.

Whitehead D. (1984). The use of an artificial urinary sphincter in irreversible urinary incontinence. *The Professional Medical Assistant* May/June, **29**, 21–30.

Wright L. (1974). *Bowel Function in Hospital Patients: The Study of Nursing Care Project Reports.* Series I, No 4. London: Royal College of Nursing.

Bibliography

Mandeslstam D. (1977). *Incontinence.* London: Heinemann Medical Books.

Wells T. (1975). Promoting urinary continence in the elderly in hospital. *Nursing Times*, **71**, (48), 1908–9.

6

Catheters and catheterization

INTRODUCTION

Catheterization is performed for a variety of reasons, such as preoperative preparation to ensure the bladder is empty, and as part of postoperative management to facilitate drainage, prevent urinary retention or provide accurate measurement of urine output in seriously ill or injured patients. It may also be used as a method of incontinence management for patients who are terminally ill and distressed by their incontinence, or for those who have intractable incontinence when all other methods have failed.

Catheterization should only be prescribed after careful consideration has been given to the situation and the merit of all other alternative actions has been examined. Indwelling catheters for the relief of incontinence should and can be avoided in many cases (Nordqvist et al, 1984); on no account should a catheter be inserted as an easy option in the management of bladder problems. The patient must fully understand the implications and give consent before an indwelling catheter is inserted.

CATHETER MATERIALS

For ease of reference catheter materials will be divided into two categories – short-term and long-term use. Catheters for intermittent or short-term use are normally made from plastic or latex, and can remain in situ in the bladder for approximately 2 weeks. Catheters for intermittent use include the Scott for females, and the Nelaton or Jacques for males. Indwelling short-term brands include Foley Simplastic. Catheters for long-term use – those which remain in situ for up to 3 months – are siliconized, teflon-coated or latex-coated with silicone elastomers or hydrogel. This process reduces the drainage lumen of the catheter. An alternative catheter for long-term use is one made from 100% silicone in which the lumen is not reduced.

LENGTH

The length of catheters varies from 20–25 cm for females to 40–45 cm for males. Unfortunately, not all professionals appear to be aware that female catheters are made, hence a number of women are catheterized with male catheters which are far too long. If one considers the difference between the male and female urethra, then the disadvantage to a female patient is self-evident. The excess tubing is either left hanging loose or else curled up and taped to the leg. If a drainage bag is to be connected to the catheter the excess length can result in the leg bag hanging below the level of the patient's hemline, unless it is curled up, which can cause kinking of the tube, obstructing the flow of urine. An ill-fitting catheter can damage the urethra and cause a stricture to form. (This will be discussed later.)

SIZE

Catheters are sized in either Charriere (CH) or French (FG) scale; these two scales are interchangeable and equate to the external circumference of the catheter as measured in millimetres. The sizes go up in even numbers from 8 to 30 FG. Catheters of 14 to 16 FG are usually the largest needed for an adult (McGill, 1982), unless haematuria or other debris is present in large quantities in which case a larger size, i.e. 18, may be required. In practice it should only occasionally be necessary to use sizes upwards of 24 FG.

Children require an 8 FG; if a smaller size is needed (e.g. in babies or infants) then a nasogastric tube is usually used. A guide to correct catheter size selection is to use the smallest size to achieve optimum drainage. In practice many professionals equate size with drainage ability and tend to use larger sizes, i.e. 16–24 FG. The use of large catheters results in greater problems with blocking and bypassing, and may traumatize the urethra (Kennedy et al, 1983). This may give rise to pressure sores and stricture formation, which can cause urine to bypass the catheter and leak out. Should this situation occur a *smaller* size of catheter is best inserted. In practice, some professionals think the reverse and insert a larger size, thus increasing the trauma to delicate urethral and bladder tissues.

The decision to catheterize a patient is usually made by the doctor. However, nurses play an important role in the decision-making process and must therefore be certain that the merits of alternative methods of managing urinary elimination have been fully explored and found wanting in the present situation. Catheterization should rarely be used as the first method of choice.

BALLOONS

Balloon catheters are marked to indicate the maximum amount of fluid the balloon will accommodate. This ranges from 3 to 75 ml. Balloon catheters for insertion into children usually have 3 ml balloons whereas the adult range includes 5, 5–10 and 30 ml and for specific post-surgical patients, 75 ml (rarely used). Ideally the smallest size balloon and catheters to allow optimal drainage should be used. In most adult patients a 5–10 ml balloon will afford effective drainage, cause less discomfort and irritation and maintain the drainage eyes of the catheter as low as possible in the bladder (Slade and Gillespie, 1985). However, many patients are catheterized with 30 ml catheters; when the balloon of this catheter is filled, it rests – like all balloons – on the bladder neck and compresses the surrounding tissues. The pressure of 30 ml of fluid can damage the delicate tissues. Another problem is due to the bladder no longer acting as a reservoir for urine whilst the catheter is in situ. This can result in the balloon becoming an irritant to the surrounding tissues and causing increased bladder contractions.

The amount of fluid used to inflate a balloon should be sufficient to keep the catheter in situ. However, this can pose practical difficulties. If, for example, a 30 ml balloon catheter is inserted, then anything less than 15 ml will cause under-inflation of the balloon. When a 5 ml balloon is used, the nurse must remember to insert 7–8 ml of fluid, as approximately 2–3 ml will remain in the tube that leads to the balloon. Water migrates through the balloon and into the bladder over a period of time so sterile water should always be used (Seth, 1986).

EYELETS AND TIPS

There are several different eyelet and catheter tip designs. The most common type is a semi-rigid round tip.

CATHETER DESIGNS

Foley catheters (balloon catheters) are familiar to nurses, and usually have a round tip, with eyelets proximal to the balloon. (Fig. 6.1A). The positioning of the eyelets does not always provide adequate drainage and leakage may occur around the sides of the urethra. If bypassing is a problem then a Roberts catheter (Fig 6.1B) with its additional eyelet below the balloon can facilitate complete emptying of the bladder, and prevent leakage. A Tiemann tip catheter (Fig. 6.1C) is often used to alleviate retention of urine in patients with an enlarged prostate gland, as the thin but firm curved tip makes its introduction into the bladder less traumatic for the patient. A Whistle tip catheter (Fig. 6.1D) may be chosen postoperatively as its lateral eyelet at the tip of the catheter facilitates drainage of blood clots, heavy haematuria and other debris which may block a catheter. Most catheter eyelets are positioned laterally or opposite each other.

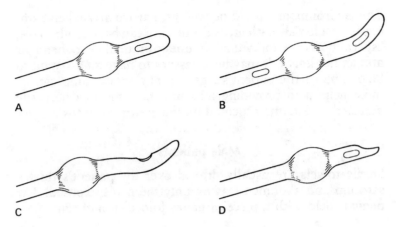

Fig. 6.1. *Catheter designs.* **A** Round; **B** Roberts; **C** Tiemann; **D** Whistle tip.

INDWELLING CATHETERIZATION

Catheterization should only be performed by a skilled practitioner. Many health authorities only allow doctors or male nurses to catheterize male patients and doctors or female nurses to catheterize female patients. In practice any competent practitioner, regardless of gender, should be able to catheterize the opposite sex if required, providing local regulations on chaperoning are adhered to and the patient has no objections. Doctors usually pass the first catheter in a male patient in case of urethral or prostatic abnormalities.

Insertion

The patient may have a catheter inserted at home or in hospital, providing an aseptic technique is used. Most practitioners are now able to avail themselves of pre-packed sterile male and female catheter packs. The contents of the packs may vary slightly between health districts, as do the procedures for catheter insertion, although the principles remain the same. If possible the patient should bathe before catheterization, or else the perineum should be thoroughly cleansed with soap and water or pre-prepared wipe. The procedure must be fully explained to the patient and consent obtained.

The environment should be well lit, particularly when catheterizing a female patient, as the urethra can be difficult to see, especially if the individual is obese or unable to bend or abduct her knees. It may be necessary to have an assistant to help support the patient's legs. An anglepoise lamp can be most helpful in providing lighting; the lamp can be easily adjusted and lighting focused on the urethral meatus.

Male patients

Sterile towels are usually draped over the patient's thighs, scrotum and abdomen leaving only the penis exposed. The penis is held with a piece of gauze folded in half (Fig. 6.2);

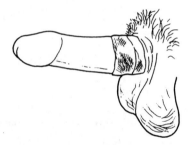

Fig. 6.2. *Position of gauze around penis.*

then the urethra and meatus are cleansed and anaesthetized with lignocaine gel. The foreskin or prepuce must be gently retracted and cleansed. At least 4–5 minutes should elapse after inserting the anaesthetic gel and before introducing the catheter in order to allow the anaesthetic to work properly.

The practitioner then puts on sterile gloves. The catheter inner package should be exposed and opened; either forceps or a gloved hand is used to pass the catheter. For ease of insertion the penis is held at right angles to the abdomen (Fig. 6.3). The catheter should be fed along the urethra without force; if an obstruction is felt, the patient should be asked to relax and take a few deep breaths. Lowering the penis to a horizontal position can often be sufficient. However, if resistance is still encountered, the catheter should be withdrawn and more lignocaine gel inserted. After a further 4–5 minutes have elapsed, the procedure for insertion should be

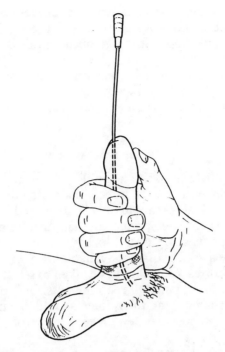

Fig. 6.3. *Position of penis for insertion of catheter.*

repeated. Some practitioners advocate the use of a smaller gauge catheter. It is always advisable to seek further advice from a urologist before proceeding.

Once urine begins to flow the balloon should be inflated with the appropriate amount of sterile water. Some catheters have pre-filled balloons which, apart from saving on the costs of needles and syringes and ampoules of water, ensure correct inflation.

The practitioner must always remember to replace the retracted foreskin.

Female patients

The perineal area is draped with sterile towels, leaving the labia exposed. A sterile receptacle is usually placed between the thighs. The labia should be separated with the thumb and finger of one hand. The vulva is then swabbed with an antiseptic solution, using downward strokes commencing at the outer labia and moving inwards (Fig. 6.4). The tip of the catheter can be dipped into lignocaine gel to facilitate meatal entry.

The balloon is inflated when urine flow commences. The catheter should then be fixed to the patient's thigh to prevent its undue movement within the urethra.

Catheter drainage bags

Once the catheter is in situ it should be attached to a drainage bag. To reduce the risk of infection a closed drainage system should be used and it should only be disturbed for an essential procedure, such as emptying the bag, instilling medication, performing a washout or unblocking the catheter.

There are a variety of bags available with fluid capacities of 350 ml to 2 litres. Care should be taken to select the one most appropriate to the patient's requirements. Only bags that have a non-return valve at their inlet should be used with an indwelling catheter, as they prevent reflux of urine into the bag.

Drainage outlet taps come in a variety of types and sizes (Fig. 6.6). Some require considerable manual dexterity to release. The urine should always be emptied into a sterile jug or at least a jug that is only used for that particular patient. It is also important not to allow drainage taps to touch the floor or any other item that might cause contamination. If correctly selected and managed, a catheter bag should last at least 2 weeks before it needs to be changed.

Emptying the drainage bag

Ideally urine should be emptied into a sterile receptacle, once the tap has been cleaned. Some procedures may involve spraying the tap with an alcohol-based spray before opening and again on closing, although there is no research to justify this action. The practitioner should wear sterile gloves to avoid the risk of contamination. If it is not possible to use a sterile jug or gloves, then each patient should have his or her own jug which must be washed and thoroughly dried after

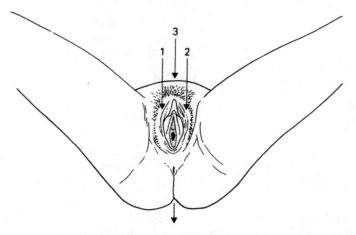

Fig. 6.4. *Swabbing the vulva before catheterization. Always swab downwards. Use a clean swab each time. Commence at the outer labia. Numbers indicate sequence of cleansing.*

each use. The practitioner should also ensure that hands are washed before and after the procedure. Great care should be taken to avoid introducing infection into the drainage system at all times. Night drainage bags are available for patients who wear a leg bag during the day.

Drainage bag supports

Drainage bags should not be allowed to hang unsupported as the downward pull may cause damage to the urethra and delicate detrusor tissue at the trigone area of the bladder. Floor-standing or bed-hanging holders are available for use when patients are in bed; these can accommodate a bag with capacity of up to 2 litres. For patients who are ambulant, a variety of holders can be discreetly worn under clothing; a 350 ml capacity leg bag is usually the most convenient type. Tapes made from Velcro, elastic, latex or fabric material may be used to secure the bag to the patient's leg.

However, not all patients find this method of support comfortable and some prefer to wear a sporran-type of catheter bag which fits around the waist. This method is not

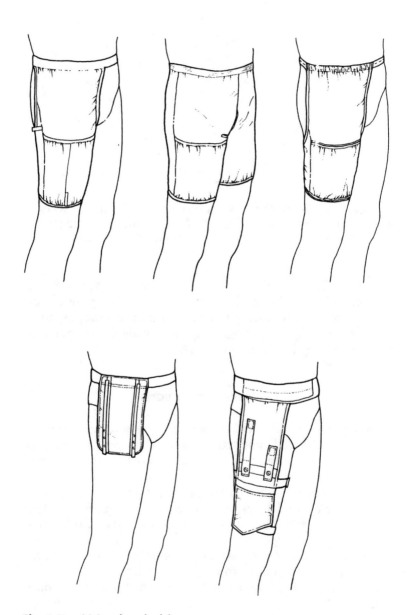

Fig. 6.5. *Urine bag holders.*

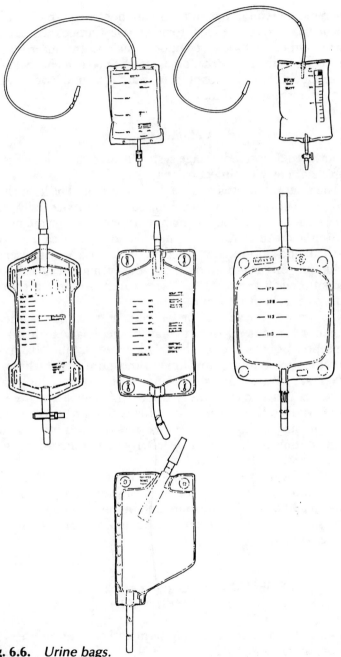

Fig. 6.6.   *Urine bags.*

always successful in patients who are obese. Alternatively leg garments or special pants, for example Cathepants, can be worn. Other methods of support include the insertion of pockets into the lining of clothes; the bag is then concealed in these pockets. It is possible to purchase underwear with pockets already sewn in.

Catheter care

Even when a closed drainage system is used there are various portals of entry for infection (Fig. 6.7).

The urethral meatus and perineal area should be kept clean and dry. The area should be cleansed at least twice daily, and after each bowel action; some practitioners favour the use of antiseptic creams around the meatus after the area has been washed and thoroughly dried. Correct use of an aseptic technique on insertion of the catheter and a closed and undisturbed drainage system with careful emptying should reduce the risk of infection.

If infection develops or encrustation of the catheter becomes a problem, then it may be necessary to instil an antiseptic solution into the bladder to inhibit bacterial growth. Noxythiolin (Noxyflex) or the more recent Clinimed Uro-Trainers are just two examples of products that have proved effective in combating urinary infections. The prevention and dislodgement of crystal formation are also possible with the appropriate Uro-Trainer and this can increase the length of time a catheter can be left in situ without it having to be changed.

Bladder washouts should not be performed routinely, and if carried out, require the same rigorous attention to aspesis. Careful and controlled introduction of fluid at body temperature is necessary to avoid trauma and unnecessary discomfort to the patient.

PROBLEMS OF LONG-TERM BLADDER CATHETERIZATION

Problems associated with long-term catheterization are well documented (Gariboldi et al, 1974; Cooper, 1977; Kunin,

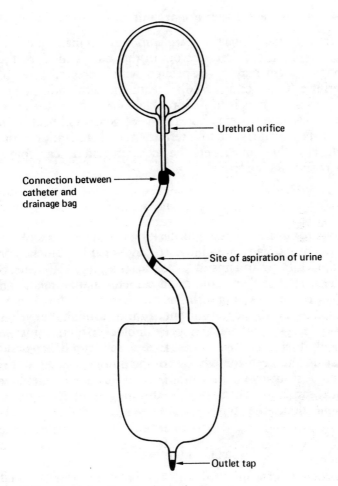

Urethral orifice

Connection between catheter and drainage bag

Site of aspiration of urine

Outlet tap

Fig. 6.7.   *Portals of entry for infection.*

1979; Bielski, 1980; Bates, 1981; Warren et al, 1981 to name but a few) and include urinary infection, urethral discomfort, renal impairment, urethral and bladder trauma and haematuria. Patients in a hospital environment are more at risk from urinary infection than those who are at home with long-term catheters in situ, due to the high number of pathogenic organisms present. In one major study it has been shown that bacteriuria developed in 44% of patients catheterized for more than 48 hours (Crow et al, 1986).

Recurrent urinary infections

Recurrent urinary infections are common for many patients with indwelling catheters. Errors in the management of the drainage system may be associated with increased rates of bacteriuria (Crow et al, 1986). Treatment with antibiotic or antimicrobial agents is futile (Brocklehurst and Brocklehurst, 1978) unless the patient shows signs of general ill health. In some instances a change to intermittent catheterization if the patient is willing and meets the required criteria can sometimes reduce the infection.

Bypassing or leakage

Reasons for urine bypassing or leaking down the sides of the urethra have already been indicated and include a blocked or ill-fitting catheter and unstable bladder (see page 110). Selecting the correct catheter and good catheter management can usually prevent this situation. The catheter may be blocked by an accumulation of debris and encrustation around the eyelets of the tube; if the catheter cannot be unblocked then it must be changed, thus augmenting the patient's self-care deficits and increasing the need for wholly compensatory nursing intervention. A study by Blannin and Hobden (1980) indicates that silicone catheters when used in the long term have fewer problems than other types.

Sexual intercourse

The presence of a urethral catheter need not inhibit sexual activity. Yet often professional carers fail to provide patients with either the opportunity to discuss their sexual needs or advice on overcoming potential or actual problems. Male patients may be advised to secure the catheter back along the shaft of the penis with tape; some partners find that sex is more enjoyable if the penis is then covered with a condom. This method is not recommended for long-term use as the friction may cause repeated trauma to the mucosa of the urethra and bladder and result in a stricture forming. Some partners find the method uncomfortable.

Female patients may prefer to be penetrated whilst lying in

a lateral position, keeping the catheter out of the way by taping it to the abdomen. Alternatively, and if practicable, the catheter could be removed before intercourse takes place. Removal could be part of the sexual act if both partners were willing. A new catheter could be inserted afterwards. Ideally catheters are best avoided in the sexually active age group and, as many 70-year-olds are sexually active, the reasons for advocating catheterization must always be explained to patients.

Suprapubic catheterization

In certain situations, such as surgical closure of the urethra (Feneley, 1983), urethral stricture or in sexually active patients who need long-term catheterization as an alternative to a urethral catheter, a catheter may be passed via the anterior abdominal wall directly into the bladder. Catheter sizes range from 6 to 16 FG. An Argyle catheter is introduced via a trocar; a Braun Cystofix catheter has a metal cannula to facilitate insertion. Some practitioners prefer to use a Foley self-retaining balloon catheter. A special flange or a suture can be used to anchor the catheter securely to the skin.

Catheter care is similar to that of a urethral catheter. A suprapubic catheter is just as easy to change as a urethral one once the channel has been established.

INTERMITTENT CATHETERIZATION

Intermittent catheterization is the term used to describe the periodic insertion of a fine non-retaining catheter into the bladder to empty it of urine; the catheter is then removed. The technique was originally used to help bladder management in patients following injury to the spinal cord as an alternative to an indwelling catheter to reduce the risk of infection and the complications associated with long-term catheterization.

The use of intermittent catheterization has now extended to other groups of patients who would otherwise be subjected to an indwelling catheter or the wearing of protective pads and pants. The use of a clean technique (Lapides et al, 1972) as opposed to an aseptic one for self-catheterization has proved to be safe and far more practical (Lancet, 1979).

INTERMITTENT SELF-CATHETERIZATION

The introduction of a clean technique for self-catheterization has done much to improve the quality of life for many incontinent patients by assisting them to meet their therapeutic self-care demands more effectively and hence reducing the amount of nursing time and the level of nursing intervention from a compensatory to an educative supportive system. Continence can be restored as the patient can empty the bladder at will, thus avoiding incontinent episodes. Retention and residual urine can be prevented, thus alleviating the risk of urinary tract infection and subsequent renal impairment.

The work of Kaye and Van Blerk (1981) highlights the effectiveness of this method of bladder management in children who have spina bifida. However, the technique is not confined to use by patients with spinal cord injury or children with spina bifida. Any patient, regardless of age, who has a bladder capacity greater than 100 ml and sufficient manual dexterity and mental ability to perform the procedure can be taught the technique (Winder, 1986). The privacy and discreetness of intermittent self-catheterization give the individual a level of social mobility and normalcy that is difficult, if not at times impossible, with other methods of bladder management.

Technique for insertion

The technique may be taught in hospital or a mutually convenient environment where the patient can be supervised until he or she becomes proficient. It may be easier for a female patient to sit in a semi-recumbent position with a mirror placed between her legs to give a good visual display of the vulva and urethra. It is possible to obtain an illuminated hand mirror or a mirror which has suction pads to keep it positioned on a toilet pan.

The perineum and urethral meatus should be cleansed thoroughly. It may be more convenient for the patient to use pre-prepared wipes. The catheter, which is usually kept in a small bag, is then removed and inserted into the bladder. Urine can be voided directly into the toilet or other appropriate receptacle. As the flow begins to diminish the individual should be taught to place a hand above the pubic bone and gently press down; this will help drain any residual urine completely. The catheter should then be removed and rinsed in cold running water to flush away any debris that may have collected in the lumen of the catheter, before being replaced in its holder until required again. Milton solution can be used to soak the catheter at convenient times.

The length of time taken by patients to become skilled at the technique will vary greatly, hence nurses must adapt their teaching strategy to maximize patient learning. Children often have great fun learning to catheterize their doll and quickly appear able to perform self-catheterization – even some 5-year-olds are quite proficient. Parents and willing teachers are also taught the method and many perform the technique for children, or supervise them until the children themselves are proficient. Carers of adult patients may also be taught the procedure.

References

Bates P. (1981). A trouble shooter's guide to indwelling catheters. *Registered Nurse*, 44, 62–8.

Bielski M. (1980). Preventing infection in the catheterized patient. *Nursing Clinics of North America*, 15, 703–13.

Blannin J. P., Hobden J. (1980). The catheter of choice. *Nursing Times*, 78, 2092–3.

Brocklehurst J. C., Brocklehurst S. (1978). The management of indwelling catheters. *British Journal of Urology*, 50, 102–5.

Cooper J. W. (1977). Urinary tract infections: causes and prevention. *Hospital Formulary*, 12, 106–9.

Crow R., Chapman R., Row B. et al (1986). *A Study of Patients with an Indwelling Urethral Catheter and Related Nursing Practice*. University of Surrey, Guildford: Nursing Practice Research Unit.

Feneley R. C. L. (1983). The management of female incontinence by suprapubic catheterization with or without urethral closure. *British Journal of Urology*, 55, 203–7.

Gariboldi R. A., Burke J. P., Dickman M. L. et al (1974). Factors predisposing to bacteriuria during indwelling urethral catheterization. *New England Journal of Medicine*, 291, 215–9.

Kaye K., Van Blerk P. J. P. (1981). Urinary incontinence in children with neurogenic bladder. *British Journal of Urology*, 53, 241–5.

Kennedy A. P., Brocklehurst J. C., Lye M. D. W. (1983). Factors related to the problems of long-term catheterization. *Journal of Advanced Nursing*, 8, 207–12.

Kunin C. M. (1979). *Detection, Prevention and Management of Urinary Tract Infections* 3rd edn. Philadelphia: Lee & Febiger.

Lancet (1979). Clean intermittent catheterizataion. *Lancet*, ii, 448–9.

Lapides J., Diokna A. G., Silber S. J. et al (1972). Clean intermittent self-catheterization in the treatment of urinary tract disease. *Journal of Urology*, 107, 458–61.

McGill S. (1982). It's the size that's important. *Nursing Mirror*, April 7, 154, (14), 48–9.

Nordqvist P., Ekelund P., Edouard L. et al (1984). Catheter free geriatric care. Routines and consequences for clinical infection, care and economy. *Journal of Hospital Infection*, 5, 298–304.

Seth C. (1986). Which catheter? *Community Outlook*, 82, 24–5.

Slade N., Gillespie W. A. (1985). *The Urinary Tract and the Catheter Infection and Other Problems*. Chichester: John Wiley.

Warren J. W., Muncie H. L. Jr., Berquist E. J. et al (1981). Sequelae and management of urinary infection in the patient requiring chronic catheterization. *Journal of Urology*, 125, 1–8.

Winder A. (1986). Intermittent self-catheterization. *The Professional Nurse*, 2, (2), 58.

Bibliography

Burgener S. (1987). Justification of closed intermittent urinary catheter irrigation/instillation: a review of current research and practice. *Journal of Advanced Nursing*, 12, 229–34.

Catheterization and Urinary Tract Infection (1983). Nursing, 2, (suppl), 13.

Champion V. L. (1976). Clean technique for intermittent self-catheterization. *Nursing Research*, 25, 13–18.

Fay J. (1978). Intermittent non sterile catheterization of children. *Nursing Mirror*, 146, xiii–xv.

Gould D. (1985). Management of indwelling urethral catheters. *Nursing Mirror*, 161, 17–20.

Hartman M. (1978). Intermittent self-catheterization. *Nursing*, 78, 72–5.

Hilton P., Stanton S. L. (1980). Suprapubic catheterization. *British Medical Journal*, 281, 1261–3.

Johnson A. (1984). *Guidelines for the Management of the Catheterized Patient*. Bard.

Pearman J. W. (1976). Urological follow-up of 99 spinal cord injury patients initally managed by intermittent catheterization. *British Journal of Urology*, **48**, 297–310.

Smart M., Ali N. (1980). Long term indwelling catheters – questions nurses ask. *Nursing Times*, **76**, 107–15.

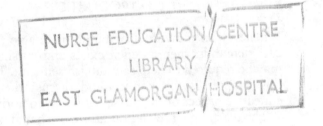

7

Teaching the patient and family self-care

INTRODUCTION

Whenever an individual or family is unable to meet health care demands, then a deficit exists and nursing intervention may be required to help re-establish self-care. The purpose of this chapter is to examine and discuss the teaching and educative aspect of the nurse's role in promoting self-care.

The teaching strategies discussed are based on the assumption that education can have a positive influence on an individual's behaviour by enhancing knowledge or skill or effecting a change in attitude. The majority of practising nurses have received very little preparation for their teaching and educative role and many lack the relevant knowledge and the opportunity to practise their teaching skills (Carter, 1981). The introduction of the English National Board Course 998, *Teaching and Assessing in Clinical Practice*, should help rectify this in the future.

PROMOTION OF HEALTH

Health education, like general education, is concerned with change in the knowledge, feelings and behaviour of people. In its most usual form it concentrates on developing such health practices as are believed to bring about the best possible state of well-being. In order to be effective, its planning methods and procedures must take into consideration both the processes by which people acquire knowledge, change their feelings and modify their behaviour, and the factors that influence such changes (World Health Organization, 1954). In practice, teaching styles have primarily concentrated on information-giving by carers who believe it is their duty either to persuade an individual to learn new patterns of behaviour or to assist him or her to bring about the desired change through informed choice. Both these approaches have the disadvantage that they ignore the question of motivation, and take no account of the need to bring about changes in society's attitudes towards incontinence or the person who is incontinent (Coutts and Hardy, 1985).

In the past, there has been a heavy reliance by medical and nursing personnel on giving patients information in the form of instructions based on professional knowledge and expertise (Vuori, 1980; Thompson, 1983), without due consideration of the attitudes and values of the individual.

ATTITUDES AND VALUES

Most attitudes and values are formed during the formative years of life and are dependent upon a variety of influential factors. If teaching is to be effective the nurse must be aware of both his or her own and the patient's prevailing attitudes and values towards incontinence and continence promotion. It is difficult to determine the length of time required to effect a change of attitude or the influence this will have on the individual's behaviour, as this varies with individuals. Some people who are incontinent may have very negative views on continence promotion, as unfortunately do some relatives and professional carers. The nurse will, therefore, require patience and determination as well as the ability to utilize his or her professional knowledge and expertise in a manner which is deemed meaningful by the patient and relatives.

TEACHING

Teaching comprises a variety of purposeful activities designed to enable or assist an individual to learn. It is not within the scope of this text to describe in detail the processes of teaching and learning; the following information is intended to highlight pertinent areas.

Principles of teaching

It is essential that the teacher knows the patient and family and the facts about the incontinence problem in addition to being knowledgeable about continence promotion and incontinence management. Nurses who feel they lack knowledge may find it beneficial to attend a specialist course, such as the English National Board course 978, *Promotion of Continence and Management of Incontinence*.

For teaching to be effective the nurse must have a systematic approach. In practice this requires the nurse to assess when a lack of learning is or will be detrimental to the promotion or maintenance of self-care. Information must, therefore, be collected and analysed before learning needs can be determined.

The next stage of the teaching process is planning. This requires the patient and nurse to decide how best, and in what order of priority, the learning needs are to be met. (For further information and helpful guidelines, see Redman, 1975). The nurse must take into consideration the patient's or relative's willingness and ability to learn and the effect this will have on the ultimate aim of encouraging and assisting the patient to achieve optimum self-motivation and self-care.

It may be helpful to define the purpose of the teaching and the intended learning outcomes in the form of learning objectives, thus enabling the nurse and patient or relatives to have a clear understanding of each other's role. The use of short- and long-term objectives helps to sustain motivation and provide evidence of continuity of performance. This framework is similar to that described in Chapter 4 (pp. 76–8). The criteria for goal planning previously described also apply to the setting of teaching and learning objectives.

A plan of teaching should clearly indicate:

1 What the patient or relatives need to know and in what order of priority.
2 The teaching and learning objectives.
3 Factors which may help or hinder the learning process.
4 An outline of the teaching content in order.
5 The teaching methods and aids to be used.
6 The preparation required to provide optimum conditions for learning.
7 The expected learning outcome.

During the implementation of the teaching plan, both nurse and patient should regularly evaluate the teaching and learning process. A planned evaluation is of great value; it should include a review of what has already been accomplished, as well as expected achievements, areas for further development and modifications needed in the existing programme. It is often neglected and misunderstood, which is to the patient's detriment (Rankin and Duffy, 1983).

Patient and relative motivation

The nurse will need to gain acceptance and the confidence of the patient and family. Many people feel threatened by terminology which is unfamiliar to them, hence the nurse must assess the situation and decide how medical or nursing terms can be replaced by terms which will be more easily understood by the individual. Alternatively, a simple and clear explanation of the technical terminology could be given. It is important that the patient knows and believes that the learning outcomes are within his or her grasp, thus clear objectives, broken down into attainable steps (as discussed in Chapter 3), are an essential part of sustaining motivation. Praise on achievement of each step helps motivate the individual towards the next goal, as does regular feedback to the patient or relative on progress.

Presentation of information

Teaching should be a two-way process involving both nurse and patient and designed to build on the individual's experience. People vary in the amount of information they want (Eardley et al, 1975) and in the amount they retain. Evidence suggests that a proportion of information will always be forgotten (Ley and Spelman, 1967). It may, therefore, be helpful to have the key aspects of a session written down and to give them to the patient as an aide-mémoire.

The success of the teaching session can be influenced by the amount and sequence of information given. Experiments have suggested that people tend consistently to recall things which they consider to be important and which are said at the beginning of a conversation (Ley and Spelman, 1965). These findings have clear implications for effective teaching as important information is frequently given throughout the period of nurse–patient or relative interaction. In practice, the problem is not difficult to overcome and requires the nurse to structure the information into categories so that delivery consists of short, concise and clear statements in a logical sequence.

The method of delivery should encourage the patient to restructure the information. Most people remember things better if they are allowed to utilize their own system of information processing (Mandler and Pearlstone, 1966). The nurse should be able, through questioning, to assess the patient's level of understanding before proceeding to the next category.

It may be helpful to provide the patient or relative with a written handout of the main points of the teaching session if a procedure is to be followed, such as self-catheterization or pelvic floor exercises. These written notes should consist of a series of logical and progressive stages in order of occurrence. This type of format will help patients to recall information and aid their understanding.

The educational principles that I have found most helpful in teaching patients and relatives are based on the adaptation of four assumptions of adult learners, postulated by Knowles (1980):

1 Concept of the patient or relative as a learner.
2 Role of the patient's or relative's previous experience.
3 Readiness to learn.
4 Orientation to learning.

Concept of the patient or relative as a learner

People move from dependence towards increasing independence and self-care at varying rates. The expectations, patience and ability of relatives to assist the patient to achieve optimim self-care are equally varied. However, most people respond more effectively when teaching styles are socratic (a two-way process which builds upon an individual's existing experience) and facilitates the active involvement of the individual.

Role of the patient's or relative's previous experience

A greater degree of meaning is usually attached by the individual to experiences gained through some activity or involvement, as opposed to when he or she is the passive recipient of information. Hence the most appropriate teaching techniques are those which involve the individual such as discussion or demonstration followed by supervised practice. If possible, group discussions between individuals with incontinence and their relatives and those who have re-established continence can be most beneficial in some situations.

Readiness to learn

Teaching will only be effective if the individual is ready to learn. It is the responsibility of the nurse to create the optimum conditions and resources for assisting the patient or relative to develop the need and readiness to learn. This process is made easier if the health care deficits identified are assessed (as discussed in Chapter 3) for lack of patient knowledge, skill or motivation; then methods to bridge the gap can be discussed with the patient and a solution agreed.

Orientation to learning

Ideally the skills and knowledge an individual gains today should help improve the effectiveness of self-care tomorrow. In practice, the learning process is reliant upon the patient's interaction with the environment and therefore tends to be performance-centred. In reality most learning is too complex to reduce to mechanistic performances (Knowles, 1980). The nurse needs to be familiar with the patient's environment and be able to facilitate and manage interaction and environment to maximize the learning opportunities.

Conditions for effective learning

There is an increasing body of knowledge to suggest that certain conditions are more conducive to learning and the promotion of self-care than others. This includes the following:

1 The patient's recognition and acceptance of the need to learn.
2 Fostering an environment characterized by mutual respect, trust and helpfulness, freedom of self-expression, acceptance of difference of opinion and physical comfort.
3 The goals of the learning experience being perceived by patients as their goals.
4 Joint responsibility of patient and nurse for planning, implementing and evaluating a learning experience.
5 Active participation by the patient in the learning process.
6 Utilizing the patient's previous experience.
7 Patients having a sense of ownership and progress towards their goals.

Selection of teaching techniques and aids

Most of the teaching undertaken by nurses is usually on a one-to-one basis with individual patients or relatives, or in small group sessions with the patient and relatives or carers. The technique used will be determined by the material which is to be learned, the number of participants involved, as well as the personal preferences and styles of the nurse and participants. For example, a mother whose child has spina bifida and is incontinent wants information about methods of bladder management for children. The information could be taught by discussion or providing appropriate reading material, or by using audiovisual material or by a combination of methods. The mother may decide that she wishes to learn the technique of intermittent catheterization to help promote and maintain her child's continence. Appropriate teaching techniques include explanation and demonstration of intermittent catheterization; demonstration is probably best performed on a model. A video or film of the procedure could also be shown. The mother could then perform the technique on the model with the nurse supervising. After careful explanation and reassurance the nurse could catheterize the child whilst the mother observes. When the child's bladder is next to be emptied, the mother could perform the technique under the supervision of the nurse. The mother could continue to perform the procedure under supervision until both she and the nurse felt she was competent to do it without supervision.

This example incorporates three types of learning – cognitive, affective and psychomotor. *Cognitive* learning refers to the acquisition of knowledge and the thought processes required to utilize the newly acquired information. The mother had to assimilate and understand the information, then demonstrate her ability to apply the knowledge in practice. *Affective* learning is characterized by the attitudes, values, beliefs and emotions which accompany any act or action and is important in the motivation of an individual to learn. The mother in our example was motivated and willing to learn how to catheterize her child to promote continence. *Psychomotor* learning refers to the acquisition of a motor skill; in the present example this was catheterization. However, in psychomotor continence promotion and incontinence management, the skills that are learnt and perfected are quite varied and determined by the ability and motivation of the individual to learn.

The nurse should always consider if the proposed teaching strategy or aid will:

1 Be acceptable and aid the patient's or relative's understanding, interest or motivation.
2 Facilitate transference of learning from one situation to another and contribute to the patient's goals or objectives.
3 Take account of the patient's and relative's age, experience and learning abilities.
4 Be flexible to accommodate the changing demands of the situation, easily available and cost-effective.

The concept of self-care means that the individual's views and abilities take precedence over the attitudes and beliefs of the professional carers. Thus patients may assume the responsibility for decisions and action which were previously undertaken on their behalf by professional carers. The change of emphasis from a professional-centred approach to a patient-centred approach may require a greater amount of the nurse's time than would otherwise be required until the patient becomes proficient and confident in taking action based on health care decisions.

HEALTH EDUCATION AND THE PREVENTION OF INCONTINENCE

Over recent years health education has, in theory, gone far beyond an approach that seeks to improve health by changing individual behaviour without taking into account the environment which enables or reinforces the possibilities of such change. Health education has come a long way from just 'blaming the victim' to a concept of developing awareness of health and providing opportunities for more informed choices to assist the individual to promote and maintain self-care skills (World Health Organization, 1981).

However, much remains to be done within the community to alleviate the distress and improve the quality of life for many people with incontinence. Nurses can do much to challenge the negative attitudes that are often present when incontinence is mentioned.

As yet there is very little media coverage about incontinence or continence promotion, other than in the professional journals. The subject is rarely acknowledged by the general media, and the topic is taboo as a subject of conversation in many social circles. With perseverance and pressure from within the community, greater public awareness of the causes and preventive aspect of incontinence, combined with information about treatments and methods to promote continence and manage incontinence more effectively may be fostered to enable individuals and their carers to make informed choices.

Ideally health education should be on a continuum commencing in the formative years and continuing until the end of the individual's life span. Elimination practices conducive to the health and well-being of the individual can be encouraged and learnt in childhood.

During pregnancy, childbirth or ill health, additional information may be required to promote and maintain continence (developmental or health deviancy self-care). Occasionally primary prevention fails to maintain the individual's normal pattern of elimination and further information is then required to enable informed choices to be made about action to facilitate early detection and treatment of the symptom (secondary prevention). If the individual becomes incontinent then the educative process should concentrate on providing information to avoid complications arising (tertiary prevention), and to re-establish continence.

Not all individuals establish or regain continence and therefore information is needed to enable them to maintain self-care. This may be provided in the form of leaflets, posters, audiovisual material, radio or television broadcasts, discussions and debates, demonstrations and the like.

SUMMARY

Effective teaching occurs in an environment which is supportive, non-judgemental and unhurried (Coutts and Hardy, 1985). However, even when the climate is conducive to learning and the patient is motivated, the acquisition of new knowledge and skill can be a difficult and, at times, painful experience. The provision of regular feedback and counselling to patients can help them more readily to accept the responsibility for meeting their self-care demands (Rankin and Duffy, 1983).

References

Carter E. (1981). Ready for home? *Nursing Times*, 77, 826–9.
Coutts L. C., Hardy L. K. (1985). *Teaching for Health – The Nurse as Health Educator*. London: Churchill Livingstone.
Eardley A., Davies F., Wakefield J. (1975). Health education by chance. The unmet needs of patients in hospital and after. *International Journal of Health Education*, 18, 19–25.

Knowles M. (1980). *Modern practice of adult education – from pedagogy to andragogy* (revised). Cambridge, New York: The Adult Education Company.

Ley P., Spelman M. S. (1965). Communications in outpatients setting. *British Journal of Social and Clinical Psychology*, 4, 114–16.

Ley P., Spelman M. S. (1967). *Communicating with the patient*. London: Staples Press.

Mandler G., Pearlstone S. (1966). Free and constrained concept: learning and subsequent recall. *Journal of Verbal Learning and Verbal Behaviour*, 5, 126–31.

Rankin S. H., Duffy K. L. (1983). *Patient Education – Issues, Principles and Guidelines*. London: Lippincott.

Redman B. K. (1975). Guidelines for quality of care in patient education. *Canadian Nurse*, 71, 19–21.

Thompson I. E. (1983). Theoretical models of health education. Appendix 1 in: *Health Education In Service Training Needs of District Nurses, Health Visitors and Midwives*. Edinburgh: Scottish Health Education Group.

Vuori H. (1980). The medical model and the objectives of health education. *International Journal of Health Education*, 19, 18.

World Health Organization (1954). *First Report of the Expert Committee on Health Education of the Public*. Technical report series No. 89. Geneva: WHO.

World Health Organization (1981). *Regional Programme in Health Education and Lifestyles: Regional Committee for Europe, Thirty First Session, Berlin, 15–19 September, EUR/RC31/10*. Copenhagen: WHO.

Bibliography

Jarvis P. (1983). *Professional Education*. Beckman. London: Croom Helm.

Levin L. S. (1973). Patient education and self-care, how do they differ? *Nursing Outlook*, March, 21, 170–5.

Pohl M. L. (1965). Teaching activities of the nursing practitioner. *Nursing Research*, 14, 4–11.

Redman B. K. (1980). *The Process of Patient Teaching in Nursing*, 4th edn. St Louis, Missouri: CV Mosby.

Rogers C. (1969). *Freedom to Learn*. Columbus, Ohio: Merrill.

Simonds S. K. (1977). Health education today: issues and challenges. *Journal of School Health*, December, 47, 10, 584–93.

Strenhlow M. S. (1983). *Education for Health*. London: Harper Row.

8

Long-term care in the community

The notion of self-care or family care to meet individual needs is not new, although greater emphasis and public awareness of this concept and its implications for the provision of care have occurred in the last two decades. This is reflected in many government documents and policy statements, such as DHSS (1981), *Care in the Community*.

Neither the psychological and sociological consequences of incontinence nor the effects on those who often heroically struggle within the community to cope with the problems that this condition frequently creates should ever be under-estimated (Tattersall, 1985). Unless adequate help and support are provided to assist individuals and their families to meet the demands made on them, they may reach breaking point, which often results in a reduction or cessation of self- or family care.

The aim of this chapter is to provide a brief overview of the methods available to avoid or minimize the risk of family crisis. By adopting a planned and systematic programme of professional intervention, and the effective use of statutory and voluntary services, the burden and isolation so often felt by individuals and their carers can be greatly reduced.

Ideally, the individual or informal carer should feel part of a wider caring network whose services to help and advise should be available to meet individual requirements.

CONTAINMENT METHODS

There are numerous aids to help contain incontinence. However, the need to select an aid appropriate to the type and severity of incontinence and the ability of the individual to use it properly is of paramount importance if containment is to be achieved. In order best to advise the patient, the nurse needs to have knowledge of the following:

1 The range and availability of aids.
2 The type and severity of the incontinence (whether urinary or faecal or both).
3 The physical and mental ability of the patient to engage in self-care.
4 The individual's lifestyle and home environment.
5 The willingness, availability and ability of carers to provide the care and assistance required.
6 The family's financial constraints.
7 The level of support and help available from statutory and voluntary bodies.

Range and availability of aids

The proliferation of products to contain incontinence has made it increasingly difficult for professionals and members of the public to decide what is the most appropriate aid to use and where it can best be obtained.

The Association of Continence Advisors has compiled the *Directory of Aids*, which they periodically update. The directory is not intended to be an exhaustive list, but rather it offers a comprehensive overview of the range of products for both male and female usage. Other information includes methods and products to control odour, alarms and enuresis training, which items are available on prescription or by mail order, and relevant comments on products and suitability of use. There are also illustrations of many of the products mentioned.

The Disabled Living Foundation also offers a valuable source of information to carers on the range and appropriateness of aids.

Pads and pants

The most commonly used method to contain incontinence is by pad and pant. All pads have an absorbent layer of material, which is usually made from wadding or wood pulp fluffed and held in shape by an outer non-woven layer of material (polyester, polypropylene, polyethylene or viscose) which comes in direct contact with the patient's skin. In addition, some pads (Tranquillity; Henleys Medical Supplies) have an absorbent gel in situ, which is designed to increase the absorbency of the pad without increasing its bulk. Many pads have a plastic backing, made from a fine-gauge polythene film, which is usually micro-embossed to reduce its contact with the skin, or else completely covered with an outer layer of material. Pads without a plastic back are relatively cheap to purchase, but need to be worn with plastic or waterproof pants which are generally quite expensive. For ease of reference, pads will be discussed under three headings, pads worn inside waterproof pants, plastic-backed pads and all-in-one systems.

Pads and the use of waterproof pants

Pads for use with waterproof pants (Fig. 8.1) come in a variety of shapes and sizes; great care should be taken to ensure the

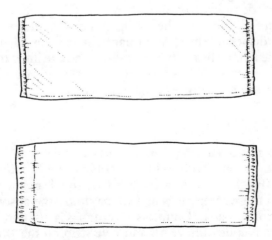

Fig. 8.1.   *Pads for use with waterproof pants.*

correct pad is used. It is practice for some patients to be provided with rolls of absorbent padding, and to cut off appropriate lengths as and when required. Although this method provides flexibility of pad size, the quality of the material uses varies considerably and many patients find the pad extremely uncomfortable. It should, therefore, not be recommended as a suitable method of containment. Despite the cheapness and trust many patients and their carers have in plastic pants, their use should, whenever possible, be discouraged owing to the potential hazard to the patient's skin. Plastic tends to cause excessive perspiration, resulting in the skin becoming hot and sticky, and thus prone to excoriation owing to a combination of perspiration, bacteria and urine. Any damage to the skin can also provide a portal of entry for bacteria and increase discomfort to the patient. In addition, frequent washing of both skin and pants are required to remove traces of unpleasant odour that can quickly form when plastic is worn in close proximity to the skin of an incontinent person. Washing tends to make the pants brittle and crack thus rendering them useless as a protective garment. Plastic also tends to rustle when the patient moves which may cause embarrassment. Much has been done to improve the design and quality of plastic pants and many pants now just have a plastic gusset, the remainder of the garment being made from other types of material. Some pants have a plastic gusset which may be separated from the skin by a pouch made of hydro-phobic material. (Urine passes through the material and into the pad). Others are disposable, i.e., Attends disposable brief. Some pants, like the confidence briefs, are made from a heavy type of plastic and are lined to prevent direct contact with the skin (Fig. 8.2); the side openings also facilitate removal and replacement of pads.

Plastic-backed pads

Plastic-backed pads come in a variety of shapes and sizes, for example, Ancilla (wing-fold) or Molnlycke's Tenaform range of pads (Fig. 8.3). These are shaped to provide greater comfort between the wearer's legs and to maximize the absorption of urine. Some pads (Cumfries; Vernon Carus and Regard; Smith & Nephew) have an adhesive strip on the waterproof backing to help keep the pad in position. Others, like the LIC

Daisy pad, have a non-slip foam strip and elasticated edges which form a dish shape to give a snug fit.

All plastic-backed pads are designed to be worn inside stretch pants. The pad should fit snugly next to the individual's skin. Patients who wish to wear their own undergarments should be encouraged to put them on top of the stretch ones, as many types of ordinary pants do not hold pads sufficiently firmly and leakage may occur. Some stretch pants are designed to be worn with specific sizes or types of pad.

All-in-one systems

All-in-one containment systems are based on the disposable nappy concept and are often referred to as diapers (Fig. 8.4). Not all professionals or patients and their carers like the term diapers; neither do they like the shape of the all-in-one garments as they equate them with the wearing of nappies and find this degrading. The garments also tend to cause the patient to perspire excessively. However, in some situations

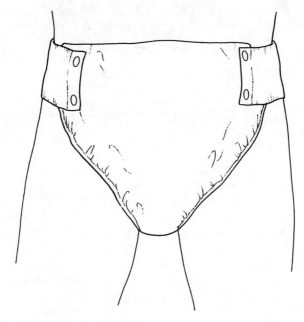

Fig. 8.2. *Confidence briefs.*

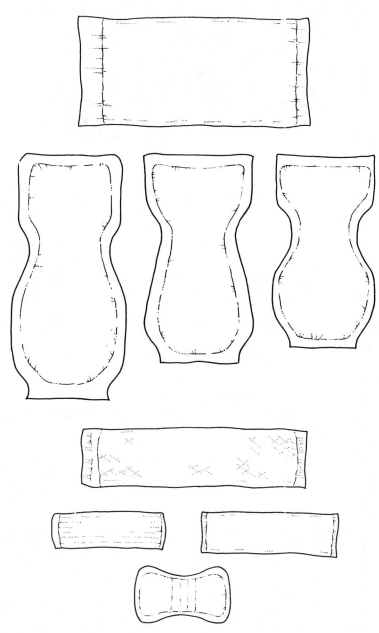

Fig. 8.3. *Incontinence pads.*

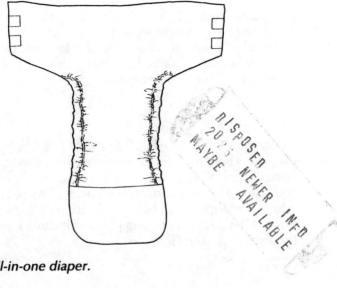

Fig. 8.4.   *All-in-one diaper.*

the pads have proved to be very effective and acceptable to the patient.

As yet, pads and pants are not available on prescription. Most patients, if known to be incontinent, usually receive a supply from their health authority often via the district nursing service. However, it is not practicable for a health authority to keep a large range of products and most stock only two or three. It is important that a range of pads should be available to meet the needs of most patients with light, medium or heavy incontinence. Nurses can do much to influence the purchase of appropriate garments by ensuring that information on products, their known performance and patients' needs is channelled to the right people, for example, supplies officers, user group representatives, chemists and senior managers. Some patients may select to purchase garments from the chemists or by mail order. However, as yet there is no central body responsible for controlling or specifying the quality of incontinence products; consequently, some patients waste money on inappropriate and poor quality products.

Male appliances

Many male patients prefer to wear an appliance as opposed to a pad and pant, providing they do not have a retracted penis or faecal incontinence. For ease of reference, appliances will be discussed under three headings – dribble pouches, penile sheaths and body-worn appliances.

Dribble pouches

Most dribble pouches (Fig. 8.5) are designed to accommodate the penis and scrotum and are worn with close-fitting pants or stretch briefs. The pouch contains material that is absorbent and tends to gel on contact with urine. The pouch is usually odour- and leak-proof, but will absorb only a few millilitres of urine. Manufacturers of drip pouches include Kanga Hospital Products, LIC and Coloplast.

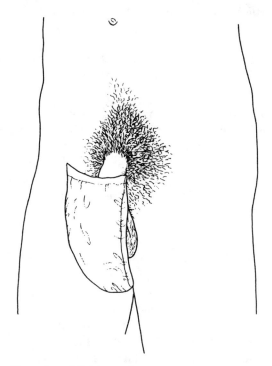

Fig. 8.5. *Tenador dribble pad.*

Penile sheaths

Penile sheaths (Fig. 8.6) are designed to be used by men with moderate to severe incontinence, or those who have frequency and urgency and are not always able to get to the toilet to void. Two types are currently available; the first consists of a one-size thin soft latex sheath that is gathered to form a rigid distal outlet; it often has a form ring at the outlet to prevent pressure and friction on the penis. The other type is made of thicker latex and therefore is less flexible, although it comes in a range of sizes and has a reinforced outlet tube and distal end. Both types are designed to be connected to a urine collection bag and may be worn either continuously or intermittently.

Some patients rely on having the correct sized appliance to keep the sheath in position. However, this is only suitable for men who are non-ambulant, and the majority of males prefer the security of some method of fixation. Some sheaths are already packaged with their own fixative and instructions for

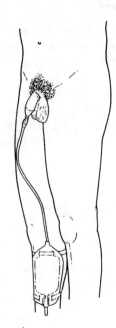

Fig. 8.6.   *Two-piece sheath system.*

use; others may recommend a method of fixation. There are three main methods:

1 Double- or single-sided adhesive foam strips which are attached directly around the penis and/ or sheath.
2 Latex or foam strips secured by some form of fastener.
3 Medical adhesive or glue – this possibly gives the securest fixation. Types include Thrackray Aquadry Medical and Dow Corning.

Patient sensitivity must be ascertained before the choice of fixative is decided.

In practice, if adhesive is used it is more effective to apply it midway down the penile shaft. Measuring and fitting instructions should be read and carefully followed and the effectiveness of the appliances monitored and evaluated at regular intervals. The patient's skin should be examined for signs of excoriation.

Body-worn appliances

Body-worn appliances have become less cumbersome over recent years, although they are still expensive and require the patient to be carefully measured and fitted. If the patient is allergic to rubber a plastic type may be worn. Ideally the patient should have two appliances.

Two main types are available. Firstly there are drip-type urinals, which collect between 50 and 100 ml of urine. These consist of an elasticated waist band and groin straps which help to keep the penile sheath and urine collecting bag in position; a scrotal support is also a feature of this type of urinal.

Secondly there are pubic pressure devices (Fig. 8.7), available in 16 sizes. These consist of a flange which fits snugly over the penis and is held against the pubis by a waist band and two leg straps. The cone is either straight (for non-ambulant patients) or curved (ambulant patients). The cone top is a secure sheath which when fitted contains the penis, with no risk of leakage. The patient or his carer must have sufficient dexterity and mental agility to clean and attach the different parts. The urine is voided into a collection bag, which may be attached to the patient's leg or placed in a hanging receptacle. Some appliances have a diaphragm instead of a pubic plate. Others include a scrotal support; those with both penile and scrotal attachments are useful for men who have a very small or retracted penis.

Most body-worn urinals are available on prescription.

Bed protection

Wet beds cause considerable personal distress and additional work and expense to the patient and family. There are various ways to protect the bed, starting with the correct selection and application of incontinence garments (although some may still leak when the patient lies prone for a prolonged period) to the use of waterproof mattress covers and drawsheets, or disposable or reusable bedpads. Mattress covers are available in various grades and sizes and offer protection for the whole bed. The main disadvantage is that they tend to make the

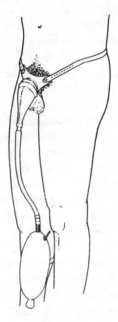

Fig. 8.7. *Body-worn male urinal.*

patient hot and uncomfortable. Some are also very noisy. All covers must be regularly cleaned to remove traces of odour. Drawsheets may be re-usable or disposable and are designed to fit across the middle third of the bed. If a plastic sheet is used and covered by a re-usable drawsheet, then laundry facilities must be considered. The plastic sheet must also be wiped clean at least once a day, and whenever it is soiled. Manufacturers of disposable drawsheets include Molnlycke, Ancilla (UK) and ACS Medical. The main disadvantage of drawsheets is that they may become displaced if the patient is restless.

Underpads are designed to be used by patients with only slight leakage of urine, or by those with faecal incontinence. However, some patients use them as a back-up to a body-worn garment in case of leakage. In practice, underpads are frequently misused by carers, especially nurses who tend to use several pads at a time for patients with moderate to heavy incontinence. Many health authorities must also share the responsibility of this misuse as some tend to purchase only poor quality pads, which are incapable of absorbing anything other than a few millilitres of urine. Good quality underpads are readily available (for example, Smith & Nephew Polyweb, Ancilla Bedpad) and usually prove to be more cost-effective than the cheaper types. Purchasers of pads should take account of the costs to the patient of unnecessary suffering due to poor quality cheap pads.

Some patients with moderate to heavy incontinence and their carers prefer to use reusable underpads or sheets. The purchase price of these protective items varies between £10 and £20. However, if properly used and providing the patient has adequate laundry facilities, they are a very comfortable and cost-effective method of containment.

Reusable underpads can be described under two headings – those which are designed to be used in conjunction with a plastic drawsheet or bedsheet and those which have their own waterproof backing. The former include Undercover Products' Hygi Everdin sheet, Nicholas Laboratories' Kylie Absorbent sheet and J. H. Bounds' Marathon Dri Sheet. The latter style includes the Ganmill Unipad, ACS Absorb Plus, Brinmark's Tri-Comfort and Domeins Confidence sheet. Urine passes through the sheet without being absorbed, so that the patient has a comfortable and dry area on which to lie. The urine is usually soaked up by the underneath layers which are not in contact with the patient's skin.

Most of these types of sheets are not suitable for patients who have faecal incontinence. The sheets tend to be rather heavy when contaminated with urine and often difficult for a frail carer or patient to handle.

Research and development into better and more effective methods to contain incontinence are taking place, hence new and improved products will be constantly appearing. The nurse is responsible for having up to date knowledge about these developments and their implication for practice.

It is not feasible to mention all the different products currently available and exclusion of some in favour of others merely reflects my personal clinical knowledge tailored to indicate the range and type of aid. Other practitioners may use different examples. However, in practice it should be the patient in conjunction with the carers who decides what will be used.

Type of incontinence and the selection of aids

The aim of any nursing intervention should be to promote patient independence and self-care, hence there is no value in advising or helping a patient to select an incontinence aid that has not been specifically designed with this aim in mind. If leakage occurs it may undermine the patient's often already low esteem and morale, in addition to increasing what may be a heavy workload for either patient or carer or both. Selection of an appropriate aid can take time and may only be achieved by a process of experimentation before one that meets the individual's personal requirements is found.

Many products indicate if they are suitable for light, moderate or heavy urine or faecal incontinence. Unfortunately, despite the proliferation of aids, there remains a dearth of good quality research to support or refute claims made by manufacturers. This makes it more difficult to advise patients or professionals on their suitability in various situations. The International Standards Organization and the British Standards Institution now draft technical standards for incontinence aids. Many small-scale trials are conducted in various situations but often their findings go unacknowledged or are inconclusive.

However, even when large-scale trials are conducted (Malone-Lee et al, 1983; Smith, 1985; Fader et al, 1986), the findings, whilst valid and reliable, can quickly become outdated as new materials and aids are introduced. There is a need for continous research and appraisal of all new products. In practice, advice and choice of aid are often based upon an individual's personal experience or expected performance. Ideally, a product should do the job for which it was intended – contain leakage of urine, faeces or both – in other words, it must be reliable (Fader and Budden, 1987). Patient confidence is also helped if unpleasant odours are neutralized or prevented from escaping, consequently many garments now incorporate deodorants. Regardless of the type or severity of incontinence or the size of the aid, it should be comfortable to wear and protect the surrounding skin from excoriation. In addition it should be easy for the patient or carer to fit and manage as well as being cost-effective.

Physical and mental ability

The physical and mental ability of a patient to engage in self-care is an important factor when selecting incontinence aids. Some patients with mobility problems experience difficulty in positioning pads (such as wing-fold) or in pulling pants up or down. Such problems can be overcome by using alternative types of pads or pants which have either side or front openings, or by assistance from carers. Impairment of an individual's mental function may preclude the use of certain types of containment garments, especially when the patient has a tendency to fiddle with or remove them.

If an indwelling catheter is being used care must be taken to ensure that the patient or carer is able to perform catheter care and operate the outlet tap on the urine collection bag. It is helpful if the nurse can observe the patient or carer perform these functions. The type of tap he or she finds easier should be the bag of choice, rather than automatically recommending the collection bag currently in use within a particular area.

Some body-worn appliances require the patient or carer to

have a good level of visual acuity and mental dexterity if they are to be properly used and a high standard of personal hygiene maintained.

Self-catheterization as a method of bladder management is usually only successful if the patient has the appropriate cognitive, affective and psychomotor skills.

Lifestyle and home environment

As incontinence becomes more widely talked about, people should become knowledgeable about products that contain incontinence in those unable to regain continence. An increasing number of incontinent people are gaining the confidence to re-establish their social lives and engage in pursuits hitherto ignored. Hence more people are becoming interested in the range of aids available. Many who wear pads and pants, for example, want to know about pad absorbency rates and methods of disposal. Not all pads are easily disposed of and many public conveniences have only small sanitary bins in the female toilets; often there is no receptacle at all in the male toilets. Instructions for disposal of appliances are usually provided by the manufacturer. However, not all toilets have the capacity to cope with soiled pads. The advice of a plumber on this issue is helpful, although often difficult for the patient and relative to seek as they may feel very embarrassed about discussing such personal problems. Some patients are extremely worried about smelling of stale urine or faeces and require a lot of reassurance, hence the value of appliances that contain a deodorant. In addition, chemists stock different types of odour controllers and their advice can also be sought. Ideally, the appliance or aid should be discreet, reliable and provide maximum comfort and independence.

The facilities available in a patient's home to manage the consequences of incontinence or to promote continence vary considerably. In the majority of cases most situations can be improved. Repeated episodes of uncontained incontinence can cause furniture and carpets to become heavily soiled and the atmosphere heavy with the unmistakable smell of stale urine or faeces, which is a source of great embarrassment to many incontinent people and their carers. Appropriate selection of aids can prevent or minimize leakage and odours can be neutralized by an airspray or by wiping furniture with, or washing clothing in, an appropriate neutralizer. Examples include Nilodor by Loxley Medical, Oxium or Chironair by Downs Surgical or Vaportak by Franklin Medical, to name but a few. Unfortunately if the fabric or furniture has become heavily contaminated, then replacement may be necessary.

Laundry facilities suitable for normal domestic use may be inadequate to cope with increased demands due to incontinence. Not all patients have a washing machine and tumble-drier and some are even without running hot water, hence the problems of even slight incontinence which requires a change of clothing or bedding can be quite considerable for some. Space to dry wet washing may be limited and on wet days washing may encroach on the living areas when it is drying. Some patients or their carers also suffer from problems of mobility or limited dexterity, so experience difficulties with wringing or pegging out washing. The use of re-usable bedsheets or pads may be precluded if the patient lacks the appropriate washing facilities or the ability to handle the soiled or wet aid without assistance. (The provision of help and support by professional and voluntary services will be discussed later.)

It is possible to purchase protective covers for chairs. However, not everyone feels comfortable being seated in a chair with a protective cover and the subject needs to be tactfully approached and discussed. Alternative methods of disposal rather than flushing soiled incontinence pads down the toilet may be required. Some patients wrap the pad up in old paper and place it in a strong plastic bag either for collection with the normal household rubbish or by a special collection service operated by the local authority. Many patients do not favour the latter as they feel embarrassed and uncomfortable that neighbours may know of their incontinence. Problems can also arise with the former method of disposal as rubbish is usually collected weekly; if bags are left outside they may be torn open by dogs or cats and their contents spilled out, which can also be a source of embarrassment and a potential health hazard. Alternatively, if left indoors, finding an appropriate space is equally if not more problematic. Storing used pads outside in a heavy-duty well sealed plastic bag placed in a bin or protected area is usually the most appropriate action.

Carers

The notion of self- and family care is implicit in many Government policy statements on health and welfare. However, little attention appears to be paid to the willingness, availability, or ability of individuals to care for their relatives. The Equal Opportunities Commission (1980) and the National Council for Single Women and their Dependants (1977) both provide evidence of the heavy emotional and physical burden which can be experienced by people caring for dependants. Many carers are themselves frail and elderly and most informal care is provided by female members of the family, usually the patient's daughter. Some carers who give up paid employment to look after a relative may be entitled to an invalid care allowance, providing the relative is in receipt of an attendance allowance. Married women who are 60 before 22 December 1984 may also be entitled to this benefit following a European Court Ruling.

Even when individuals are willing to care for relatives, they may be lacking the confidence or skill to perform all the required tasks, and some may feel embarrassed or ill at ease when assisting their relative with toileting or hygiene activities. The patient may feel equally awkward and prefer not to have the relative present, especially if it involves him or her seeing or washing soiled garments or skin. The nurse needs considerable tact and diplomacy to elicit the views of both patient and carer about the limits of care. By involving, supporting and listening to the views of both carer and patient many potential crisis situations can be avoided or the effects minimized.

The extent of involvement by carers to meet health care needs varies according to the individual patient's ability to maintain self-care. Some require almost constant help to maintain continence or manage the consequences of incontinence. The longer a person remains soiled or wet, the greater the discomfort and risk of skin excoriation, odour formation and leakage.

Regimes to promote continence may have to be adjusted to

fit in with the presence of the carer. Techniques to re-educate or train the bladder may require the help of the carer, either to assist or remind the patient to go to the toilet. Sometimes careful selection of aids or appliances can reduce the involvement and physical effort of the carer. For example, the patient may with training be able to use a walking aid or learn to respond to an alarm to remind him or her to go to the toilet. Carers can be taught good safe lifting and transfer techniques, thereby reducing the strain often felt by themselves and the patient during these activities.

In some situations mechancial lifting devices can be most helpful, although most take up too much space for the average house. Bathing seats or stools such as the Bathability by Warren Hooker (Fig. 8.8) can help the patient maintain good personal hygiene. Sometimes the installation of shower facilities makes washing much easier. However, some elderly people do not like the idea of a shower. Cost can also preclude their installation.

The availability of relatives to care should be assessed carefully, as many potential carers have other dependants to look after and some are also in paid employment on a full- or

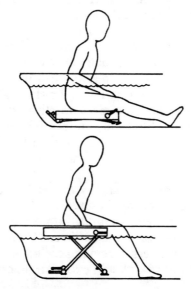

Fig. 8.8. *The Bathability (Warren Hooker).*

part-time basis. If asked or expected to become heavily committed to caring for an incontinent relative, many become over-tired and stressed, which can cause tension within the family unit.

Often carers are expected to perform tasks at home when they have not had any training or instruction, such as would be given to student nurses if the patient was in hospital. During home assessment nurses should assess any skill or knowledge deficits which the carer or patient may have and which may reduce the quality of care given. Deficits may be overcome and confidence increased by providing the individual with the opportunity to acquire the appropriate knowledge and skill to achieve pre-determined realistic goals. The setting of goals or objectives is a useful method of assessing the progress of individual carer and patient. A date and time should always be given when both carer and patient can separately and jointly give their opinions on the effectiveness of the care provided, and the changes they think are required to enable the patient to maintain optimum independence and self-care.

Carers may find additional help and support from the Association of Carers, First Floor, 21-3 New Road, Chatham, Kent ME4 45Q (Tel: 0634–81398), or other voluntary caring bodies, many of whom offer emotional support and practical help and advice. It is not acceptable practice to assume that relatives are coping with the incontinence problem just because they do not seek professional help or advice. It is the responsibility of the professional carers to ensure that those who are less qualified receive adequate support so that there is minimal disruption to the lives of the patients, carers and their families.

Financial constraints

Incontinence can necessitate increased expenditure, which on a fixed low income may result in financial hardship for the incontinent person and family. Failure to disclose incontinence to the appropriate professionals usually means that the patient does not receive appropriate assessment and advice on continence promotion or the most effective methods to contain the incontinence. In these cases, many people resort to

the private purchase of often expensive and sometimes inappropriate aids and appliances. Some are not even aware
that several items, such as pads and pants, can be provided
free of charge and that others are available on prescription
(male body-worn appliances, for example). Leakage of urine
can wet the patient's under and outer clothing, bedding or seat
covers, producing large quantities of washing. The cost of
washing powder, electricity and hot water can be high over a
period of time, further draining limited resources. Repeated
washing also shortens the life of garments and bedding,
necessitating expensive replacements.

Support from statutory and voluntary bodies

The level of support provided to patients and informal carers
by voluntary and statutory bodies varies between different
health districts. Often patients with additional disabilities
receive greater support than those whose main symptom is
incontinence. Some authorities operate a free delivery and
collection service for certain incontinence items (pads, pants,
bed- or drawsheets). A laundry service for those with incontinence is also provided in some districts; the frequency of
collection and delivery varies. Those which operate on a
weekly basis can leave the heavily incontinent person short of
personal clothing and bedding. Occasionally a linen loan
service is available to help patients overcome this difficulty. It
may be possible for a patient without a washing machine to
have one on loan from the social services. In areas where no
laundry service is operated considerable hardship can be
experienced; this may result in a request for the patient to
enter into residential care.

Some patients may qualify for meals-on-wheels or home
help. Numerous organizations like the British Red Cross, St
John Ambulance, Age Concern, and the Women's Royal
Voluntary Service offer emotional support and practical help
and advice to those in need.

The involvement of the community occupational therapist
and physiotherapist is essential if the patient is to receive
expert advice on aids and exercises to promote and maintain
self-care. While the short- or long-term loan of aids to assist in
toileting and personal hygiene are invaluable, others prefer

the opportunity to select and purchase their own appliances after being given advice and information. It may be possible to obtain financial help from the DHSS to meet additional expenditure or to replace worn out items.

Nurses need to find out the range and extent of the services available within their own district, and how the patient can obtain those which are relevant to help maintain independence.

References

Association of Continence Advisors (1988). *Directory of Incontinence and Toileting Aids.* London: Disabled Living Foundation Information Service, 380–84 Harrow Road, London W9 2HU.

Equal Opportunities Commission (1980). *The Experience of Caring for Elderly and Handicapped Dependants/Survey Report.* Manchester: EOC.

Fader M., Budden G. (1987). Coping with incontinence garments. *Pharmacy Update*, July–August, 3, 207–73.

Fader M. J., Barnes K. E., Malone-Lee J. et al (1986). *Incontinence Garments: Results of a DHSS Study.* Health Equipment Information No. 159. London: HMSO.

Malone-Lee J., McCreery M., Exton-Smith A. N. (1983). *A Community Study of the Performance of Incontinence Garments. Aids Assessment Programme.* London: DHSS.

National Council for Single Women and their Dependants (1977). *The Impact of Caring.* London.

Smith B. A. (1985). A comparative trial of urinary incontinence aids. *British Journal of Clinical Practice*, 39, 311–19.

Tattersall A. (1985). Getting the whole picture. *Nursing Times*, April 3, 81, (14), 55–8.

Bibliography

Association of Carers, First Floor, 21–3 New Road, Chatham, Kent ME4 5Q. (Tel: 0634–81398).

Dawson B., Wilkinson E. (1988). Ward-based comparison of two incontinence care products. *Care Science and Practice*, 6, (4), 105–6.

Egan M., Thomas T., Meade T. (1985). Mix and match. *Community Outlook*, June, 81 (24), 32–7.

King M. (1984). Aids for incontinence. *Nursing Mirror*, 158, 30–1.

Pottle B. (1986). When the sheets were changed. *Nursing Times*, November 26, 82 (48), 64–6.

Seth C. (1987). Male incontinence. *Community Outlook*, February, **83** (5), 20–1.

Timms A., O'Hara S. (1988). To investigate the existence of a bacteristatic or bactericidal effect of copper impregnated incontinence pads on common urinary tract organisms. *Care Science and Practice*, **6** (4), 109–11.

9

Special needs of the elderly, children and the disabled with problems of incontinence

There is a great need to improve the attitudes of carers and the existing level of services currently available in many areas for those who suffer from either urinary or faecal incontinence. Children, for example, are often expected to make do with poor quality aids and appliances, many of which are not designed with the needs of children in mind. Some are merely scaled down replicas of adults' aids.

At the other end of the age range urinary incontinence affects 11% of women and 6% of males over the age of 65 (Thomas et al, 1980), and in residential local authority homes for the elderly urinary incontinence is a major management problem with 16–25% of the residents frequently incontinent (Tobin and Brocklehurst, 1986b). In one study, over 10% of residents in 30 residential homes were found to have faecal incontinence at least once a week (Tobin and Brocklehurst 1986b). Unfortunately mopping up the mess is often the only course of action carers take when an elderly person is incontinent. This negative approach to management is often due to the prevailing attitude that incontinence is a factor of advancing age and therefore cannot be cured. These attitudes are often compounded if the individual, whether child or adult, has either a mental or physical handicap or both.

The aim of this chapter is to look briefly at various methods that can be used to change the negative attitudes of many patients and carers by demonstrating the positive steps that can be taken to promote continence or to manage the incontinence more effectively and thus improve the quality of life for the patient and job satisfaction for the carer.

ELDERLY PEOPLE

The key to the successful treatment or management of incontinence is good assessment and accurate diagnosis, combined with a positive and informed attitude of patients and their carers.

Detrusor instability

The majority of elderly men with detrusor instability associated with chronic retention of urine and overflow incontinence, who are otherwise physically fit, respond well to surgical intervention (Sole and James, 1984). It is however important to follow up all patients postoperatively to identify those who develop postoperative dribbling. Follow-up could be on a self-referral basis to the patient's own general practitioner or directly to any appropriate department or individual with the facilities and expertise to help the patient.

Many elderly patients with an unstable bladder after cerebrovascular accident can be helped to regain control over micturition by a combination of toilet training, anticholinergic medication (if appropriate) and rehabilitation. The success of this type of regime is greatly enhanced by effective communication between professionals, family and the patient, who must also understand the reasons for the regime and have sufficient motivation to comply (Castleden et al, 1985).

Apathy

Many elderly patients are wrongly accused of being apathetic about their incontinence. Assessment may reveal that the patient has signs of clinical depression which requires investigation and treatment. Often depression can follow a sudden life crisis such as a bereavement, an acute episode of illness or a change of environment such as long-term hospitalization or residential care, or a long-term disability (such as parkinsonism). Apathy may be the individual's attempt to cope with a distressing situation by withdrawing from that situation.

Cognitive and psychomotor skill

Age is usually accompanied by a loss of cognitive or psychomotor skills; the degree of loss varies with the individual. This will affect the elderly person's ability to practise self-care over elimination. A specific brain lesion or a confused state can compound the problems.

Careful assessment is necessary to establish the following:

1 The level of patient's awareness of the urge to void or defecate.
2 The ability to 'hold on' and to identify the toilet and get to it.
3 The ability to remove all appropriate clothing out of the way and to sit on or stand in front of the toilet as appropriate.
4 The ability to reach and use the appropriate equipment to wipe or cleanse the perineal area as required.
5 The ability to flush the toilet and to replace the articles of clothing correctly, and to wash the hands on completion of this procedure.

The assessment should also seek to establish a baseline by determining the patient's present eliminative self-care.

Planned intervention

Intervention, as discussed in Chapters 3 and 4, should be designed to meet established care needs, but in a manner which maximizes independence and self-care. If, for example, the patient has the ability to get to the toilet but lacks awareness of the need to void, then techniques to remind him or her of this need should be employed. Verbal prompts by carers are usually sufficient. However many incontinent elderly people living at home may not have the continual presence of a carer, hence pre-set buzzers or alarm clocks to act as reminders can enable a person to maintain continence. If the individual is unable to reach the toilet unaided, and help is not available, an alternative receptacle can be provided in the form of a hand-held urinal, bedpan or type of portable toilet. It is important, however, to establish who will be responsible for emptying these receptacles.

Residential or hospital care

In hospital or residential homes for the elderly it is important that the toileting regime for each patient should continue to be based on an assessment of his or her bladder patterns. It must be emphasized that bladder and bowel function should always be carried out unhurriedly and in private. Communal toilet sessions are still a familiar scene in some environments with patients often taken several at a time to the toilet and expected to void on demand. Unfortunately it is not uncommon to hear a nurse comment on a patient: 'She deliberately wet as soon as I got her back to her seat'. This type of comment reflects the lack of knowledge about the individual patient's bladder pattern and the emotional trauma that is often caused to elderly people by carers' insensitive attitudes to toileting and the basic human need to preserve dignity. Many patients are so tense during the toileting procedures that the urethral sphincters are not relaxed until they are once again seated in their chair or bed. Rushed and insensitive handling can cause agitation and even confused states in some elderly patients (Clay, 1978).

Reality orientation

Sometimes incontinence occurs because the patient cannot easily find the toilet; it may be helpful in this type of situation for easily seen signs to be erected showing the way. However, in addition, it may be necessary to reinforce verbally how to use the signs and then to observe the patient's understanding of them, as some elderly people have difficulty in adjusting to new situations due to a diminished ability of the brain to respond to different or new stimuli.

Some patients suffer from dyspraxia – they are unable to

complete a task in a logical sequence in the absence of obvious major intellectual, auditory, visual or psychomotor deficit. Although patients may know and are able to perform the skills required for toileting, they may do them in the wrong order and be inappropriately labelled as apathetic or senile, with no attempt made to promote continence. Prompts for each stage of the task can help to overcome this problem, once it is understood. However, many nurses fail to understand the need to prompt someone frequently to do something which the nurse considers to be an automatic act, with the result that this aspect of continence promotion is neglected.

Behaviour modification

In situations where most of the carer–patient contact is during mopping up procedures, the result may be reinforcement of social contact due to being wet or soiled rather than dry (Tarrier and Larner, 1983). The main aim of a behaviour modification programme in elderly confused patients is to extinguish the undesirable behaviour (i.e. the incontinence) by reinforcing the desired pattern of behaviour, i.e. to re-establish continence by voiding in the appropriate place, at the right time. It is necessary for nurses to chart the frequency and type of interaction they have with patients who are incontinent and who are going to undergo a behavioural programme. The desired behaviour can be rewarded and reinforced by a variety of methods which include praise, attention and social and physical contact during periods of continence, or when proper use of the toilet facilities is made. If the patient is incontinent then the situation should be dealt with quickly and effectively but with only essential physical and professional contact. If behaviour modification is used continuously and consistently over a period of weeks by *all* the carers, both day and night success can be achieved in some patients.

Faecal incontinence

There are few symptoms more unpleasant or distressing for both patient and carer than faecal incontinence. Yet most incidences can be prevented by appropriate diet and the development of good bowel habits. However, of those who become incontinent, most cases with good assessment and proper management can either be cured or significantly improved (Henry, 1983). Tobin and Brocklehurst (1986a) estimate that the lives of up to 10 000 residents could be improved by effective management.

Faecal continence is maintained through neuromuscular co-ordination and activity, as discussed in Chapter 2. Tobin and Brocklehurst (1986a) found that faecal incontinence, secondary to impaction and neurogenic incontinence (possibly due to the inability to inhibit defecation), occurred predominantly in elderly demented patients. Some patients who are demented lose their awareness of the social necessity to maintain continence until they are in an appropriate place – the toilet – and tend to defecate in the bed or in their clothing. A few select the nearest receptacle (such as a waste bin, a pan or the sink) and use it, much to the distress of those around them. With accurate assessment, it is possible to identify and treat as appropriate any underlying pathological causes. The behaviour of some patients changes immediately prior to elimination (they become restless, agitated or wandering) and careful assessment may enable carers to identify the 'call to stool' and give them time to assist them to get to the toilet to empty their bowels normally.

The principles of behaviour modication can also be used to promote faecal continence in some patients. Occasionally continence is not achievable, and the patient requires assistance to contain the incontinence. This may be by wearing protective garments in the form of pads and pants, or as some patients prefer, by wearing a faecal collector such as the Incare one (Fig. 9.1). A protective barrier which adheres to the patient's perineum, cleft and inner surfaces of the buttocks holds the collector firmly in situ. Either fluid or formed stools can be contained with any unpleasant odours neutralized by an odour barrier film. Most cases of faecal incontinence can be cured or improved (King, 1980).

CHILDREN

Introduction
For the majority of children, the process of learning the skills to attain continence is largely uneventful, and most children

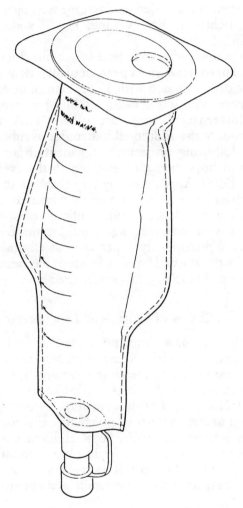

Fig. 9.1.   *Faecal collector.*

are continent of both urine and faeces by the age of 4 years. Continued wetting after the expected age of continence is termed incontinence if an organic dysfunction is present and enuresis if organic dysfunction is absent (Timmreck, 1983).

Many children acquire day-time control of their bladder before night-time control. (About 50 per cent of children are dry during the day by the age of 3 years; Meadow, 1980). The terms diurnal enuresis defines day-time wetting and nocturnal enuresis night-time bed wetting. Faecal soiling is termed encopresis.

Surveys suggest that girls tend to become drier earlier than boys and approximately 45 per cent of all girls aged between 2 and 3 are dry compared with 33 per cent of boys in the same age category (Sillitoe and Reed, 1986). Approximately 13 per cent of children aged 5 years are still wet (Lask, 1977); many have to endure the additional indignities of ridicule and even hostility following an enuretic incident. Enuresis is more common in boys than girls even up to the age of 14 years (Shaffer, 1976). Approximately 7 per cent of all boys aged 7 years suffer from enuresis compared with only 3 per cent of girls (Sillitoe and Reed, 1986). Studies suggest that enuresis diminishes with increasing age (Wishart and Bidder, 1981). However, approximately 1 per cent of all children remain enuretic by the age of 18 years. Enuresis has been highlighted as a factor of homelessness (Stone, 1983).

Causes of enuresis and encopresis

Several theories have been postulated as to the causes of enuresis and encopresis. These include genetic factors and delayed maturation of the child's nervous system (Bakwin, 1983); social class and being socially disadvantaged (Broomfield and Douglas, 1956); inadequate training and habit formation, and emotional or psychiatric disorders (Rutter et al, 1973; Simmonds, 1977). Some children are reported to have an emotional or psychological block about elimination (Robbins, 1985). Encopresis is usually associated with a stressful situation within the family (Landman and Rappaport, 1985).

Enuresis may be classified as primary when the child has not experienced episodes of continence, or secondary, when periods of continence are interspersed with episodes of wetting. Nocturnal enuresis is more common than diurnal enuresis. The latter, however, is evident to people other than the child's immediate family, and when peers are involved can be a source of even greater embarrassment and distress for the child.

Children may suffer enuretic episodes at school if they have
frequency or urgency and if the teacher will only allow visits
to the toilet at set times, hence the children who cannot 'hold
on' will invariably wet themselves. Such situations can be
further aggravated if the child is then rebuked by the teacher.
Fortunately, most teachers and parents are more sensitive and
are usually sympathetic and offer reassurance.

Intervention

Most children with diurnal enuresis will become dry without
any specific nursing or medical intervention. However,
because of the distress the symptom causes, professional
advice is frequently sought and various techniques are
employed to promote continence. The child and parents may
be advised to try techniques which will train the bladder to
hold increased amounts of urine by extending the period
between sensation to void and the uncontrollable urge to
empty the bladder if frequency or urgency is the cause of the
enuretic episodes. The techniques are similar to those already
described in Chapter 4; the child is instructed to go to the
toilet at pre-set times or gradually to extend the period
between sensation and voiding. It is important to commence
this type of intervention when both parent and child can give
adequate time to the programme; usually school holidays are
an optimum time, providing the family is not going away on
holiday.

The child should be encouraged to keep a record of progress
made. Each dry episode should be praised and the child
reassured that complete continence is achievable, even though
this may take time.

Children, like adults, can also suffer from stress incontinence. Intervention is usually a combination of pelvic floor
exercises and interruption of the urine flow mid-stream (as
described in Chapter 4). However, not all children respond to
this type of intervention and some require surgical intervention to correct anatomical abnormalities.

The type of intervention instigated for a child with nocturnal enuresis should be decided following a detailed assessment
of the child and the family situation, since much usually
depends upon parental co-operation and the relationship

between the child and parents and other siblings. Empathy and the ability to reassure the parents and child that the situation can be improved are essential prerequisites for the nurse involved. It may also be necessary in some cases to provide help for the parent or guardian with washing and drying soiled linen.

It is essential that the child should be properly assessed to exclude anatomical abnormalities and urinary tract infection; the latter can be a cause of enuresis in young girls (Kolvin et al, 1973).

Some children are afraid of the dark, and prefer to remain in bed to void, rather than get up to face the terrors of the dark. In such cases the use of a night light may be all that is required. Changes within a family, such as the arrival of a new baby, can trigger enuresis. If this is considered to be a factor, then the situation should be carefully explained to the parents and the child given ample reassurance of continued parental love and affection.

The child should be encouraged to empty the bladder before going to sleep. Some parents even restrict fluids during the evening in an attempt to prevent wetting. However, this is seldom an effective method of treatment in the long term as relapses are quite common. Some children attain continence by being awoken from sleep during the night by parents and taken to the toilet to void. In practice this method of intervention can be detrimental to the parents, as it interrupts their own sleep pattern and can give rise to tiredness. The use of a star chart (Fig. 9.2) can be effective in treating many children with enuresis within a relatively short period of time, such as 7–21 days. The idea is to encourage the child to place a star on the chart for each night he or she is dry. When three consecutive stars are achieved then the child receives a gold star, which may be exchanged for a small gift. The high level of motivation and child involvement this type of activity creates appears to contribute to the high level of success.

However, not all children attain continence using this technique, and various methods of conditioning to strengthen the child's desired response not to wet the bed and weaken the maladaptive behaviour of wetting the bed may be employed (Timmreck, 1983). The use of a bell or buzzer has proved successful for many children. If well supervised this method

Name _____   Date chart commenced _____

Don't forget to go to the toilet before you go to bed.
Put a star on the chart in the morning if you have a dry night.
For three dry nights in a row you can stick on a gold star.

Day	Week 1	Week 2	Week 3	Week 4	Week 5	Week 6	Week 7
Monday	★		★	★			
Tuesday		★	★	★			
Wednesday		★	★	★			
Thursday	★			★			
Friday		★	★	★			
Saturday	★	★	★	★			
Sunday			★	★			

Fig. 9.2.   *Star chart.*

will cure 80 per cent of bedwetters (Norton, 1986). The child
lies on a special urine-sensitive pad, which is connected to an
alarm or buzzer. The slightest drop of urine triggers the alarm
mechanism, which is designed to inhibit micturition and wake
the child so that he or she can get up to go to the toilet to
complete voiding. However, the method is not without its
drawbacks. Firstly, the child must understand what is
expected. Secondly, not all children are woken by the buzzer,
so parents need to be able to hear the buzzer and to take
appropriate action. If the child shares a room with other
siblings they may be disturbed by the noise and subsequent
activity. Thirdly, it is necessary to reset the alarm mechanism
after each use. A record of the number of times per night the
buzzer is activated and the subsequent action, including the
size of the wet or damp patch, should be made.

The period of time required before the child responds to the
alarm will vary. Unfortunately, evidence suggests that whilst
this type of technique is helpful in initially improving the
situation, there is a relatively high rate of relapse (about one-

third) (Turner et al, 1980). However, overlearning (Morgan, 1978) can reduce the number of children who experience a relapse. After attaining 14 consecutive dry nights, the child is required to increase evening fluid consumption by 0.5–1 litre, whilst still using the alarm. This may result in episodes of enuresis, but the child will quickly become continent again, and once dry for a further 14 consecutive days, the increased fluid intake should cease and the alarm be discontinued. If the child is unable to tolerate the increased fluid and continues without signs of diminution to have wet episodes during the overlearning period, the fluid intake should be reduced and the alarm system continued until he or she becomes dry again, when a further attempt at overlearning can be made.

Some children are treated using a rapid training technique, for one night (Azrin and Fox, 1974). The aim is to give children a large fluid intake, wake them every hour through the night and give them another drink, then take them to the toilet whereupon they are rewarded on each occasion they void in the toilet. This period of intense training is followed by the use of a buzzer system for 2–3 weeks. It is, however, extremely demanding for both the children and parents and does not appear to be widely advocated by professional carers.

Hypnosis can also be used to cure secondary enuresis in children over the age of 8 years. The therapy can involve the whole family and is designed to obtain a positive shift in the attitude of the enuretic child's family towards the child and the bed wetting. The evidence of hypnosis and promotion of continence is scanty, hence its full value and potential are difficult to assess. Anticholinergic drugs (for example imipramine, Tofranil) are sometimes prescribed. The drugs may be taken without other types of intervention or in conjunction with other forms of treatment, such as a star chart. Unfortunately many children suffer a relapse on or shortly after withdrawal of the drug (Blackwell and Currah, 1973).

Encopresis

Faecal soiling or encopresis is much less common than enuresis, but is often more distressing to the child's parents. However, in the absence of organic abnormalities, most children respond well to various types of intervention. As stress is frequently associated with this symptom, sensitive and thorough assessment of the child's home and social environment should be undertaken and if possible, the child should be encouraged to talk about the soiling and why he or she thinks it happens. Sometimes the child is responding to conflict within the family or is afraid to use the toilet and has developed a toilet phobia (Lask, 1977). Painful constipated motions can inhibit a child from voluntary passage of faeces, which may then result in faecal soiling due to spurious diarrhoea. Methods to alleviate and prevent constipation have already been discussed.

A star chart can also be used for children with encopresis and rewards given as for the enuretic child. Treatment is often family-centred (Landman and Rappaport, 1985). Very occasionally a severely disturbed child will smear faeces and some have been known to swallow faecal matter (coprophagia). When such situations arise, the child should be referred to a psychologist or psychiatrist for assessment.

Children and containment garments

At times it is extremely difficult to obtain good quality and appropriate sized garments or aids to contain either urinary or faecal incontinence. The wearing, disposal, or emptying of these items can be a great source of inconvenience and distress to many school-age children. If possible the school nurse should be notified when a child with incontinence is to attend 'ordinary school' so that she can discuss with the teaching staff appropriate facilities for either changing or emptying the containment garment, thus encouraging the child to be independent and confident. Promoting continence or effectively containing incontinence in children requires tact, initiative and clinical expertise if the child is to be able to maintain self-care and have independent control over bowel and bladder functions.

THE HANDICAPPED PERSON

Attitudes towards people who are handicapped may be influenced by cultural, religious or political beliefs and therefore often differ between various groups within and between societies.

A handicap may be congenital (such as spina bifida) or acquired (for example, injury to the spinal cord), and can affect the individual physically or mentally. A few individuals have both a mental and physical disability (for example, cerebral palsy).

It is difficult to give a precise definition of the term handicap, although the definition of a handicapped child can be defined as one who is suffering any continuing disability of body, intellect or personality likely to interfere with his or her normal growth, development and capacity to learn, seems very suitable.

The main types of handicap are:

1 Cerebral palsy.
2 Muscular dystrophy.
3 Multiple sclerosis.
4 Spina bifida.
5 Hemiplegia, paraplegia and tetraplegia.
6 Mental handicap.

Cerebral palsy occurs when the area of the brain responsible for controlling and co-ordinating movement and muscle tension is damaged. Muscles are either flaccid or spastic. The child often has difficulty with tasks that require manual dexterity. The extent to which the lower limbs are affected will determine whether the child can walk with aids or is confined to a wheelchair. Sometimes the child may have jerky and uncontrolled movements of muscles (athetoid movements); this is usually due to damage to the centre of balance or equilibrium within the brain. Some children with athetoid palsy may initially be very flaccid or floppy; later (after a year or so) they begin to wriggle and move almost constantly, giving the appearance of being extremely restless, often twisting and grimacing.

Unfortunately the obvious physical disabilities caused by many handicaps often result in individuals being treated as mentally subnormal, although most are of normal or high intelligence. Much is now being done by various organizations to educate people and develop ways of assisting individuals to overcome their disabilities and to be as independent as possible. Some handicaps, like the neuromuscular disorder of muscular dystrophy or multiple sclerosis which affects older children and adults, are both degenerative and progressive, although individuals with multiple sclerosis often experience long remission, sometimes extending over years, and a temporary regaining of lost functions.

Spina bifida occurs when there is a malformation of the lower portion of the spinal cord. The extent of the spinal defect varies from minor and not easily detectable to an obvious swelling (meningocele) and sometimes the spinal cord and surrounding nerve tissues are exposed (myelomeningocele). The extent of the handicap will vary with the severity of the defect; a child may be paraplegic and suffer loss of sensation and be incontinent. Most children with spina bifida are of normal intelligence.

Complete transection of the spinal cord results in either paraplegia or tetraplegia. The extent of the paralysis usually relates to the location of the transection. Paraplegia occurs following injury to the spinal cord below the level of the neck, whereas tetraplegia (when all four limbs are paralysed) occurs in lesions affecting the cervical spine and may affect the respiratory muscles. Initially the patient suffers from spinal shock, a flaccid paralysis causing the bladder and bowels to become atonic and over-distend, as sensations of fullness are not registered in the brain and spinal reflexes are absent.

Many individuals have a mental handicap without a physical handicap. However, a proportion are multiply handicapped, and require a greater level of assistance and support to enable them to achieve independence within the constraints of their disabilities.

Promoting self-care

In most situations it is usually possible to improve the existing quality of life for both patient and carer. The first priority must be to determine by careful assessment the extent of the disability. This may require developing new methods of communicating if the patient has a defect in speech, hearing, vision or understanding. The nurse must then assess the individual's potential and limits for self-care. The ability of an individual to acquire, maintain or regain continence is often a major factor in deciding where that person can or cannot live. Individuals are excluded admission to some types of residential accommodation if they are incontinent. Families' continuing willingness to care for their relative at home often hinges on the effective containment of incontinence or promotion of continence.

Toilet training

If toilet training is going to be successful in individuals with a mental handicap, then it requires persistence and co-operation from all those involved in that person's care. There are several methods of toilet training, mostly based upon the principles of behaviour modification. Appropriate behaviour (remaining dry, using the toilet properly) is rewarded in some way (praise, cuddle, small treat) and thus reinforced, whereas inappropriate behaviour (incontinence) is not acknowledged, other than ensuring that the patient is changed.

Some behaviour programmes use punishment as a means of discouraging inappropriate behaviour. Personally I consider punishment a negative and unethical act and one which should be discouraged in favour of positive reinforcement and reward.

It is important that the carers should be consistent in their approach to toilet training. It may therefore be of value if the nurse is aware of the relationships between the patient and carers. Tierney (1973) devised a useful method for establishing a good pattern of toilet behaviour in which she identified the patient baseline behaviour then set intermediate and terminal behavioural objectives.

Sometimes patients may know when they want to void, but be unable to communicate in the normal manner to the carers. The nurse or carers should observe the individual for changes in behaviour which might indicate the desire to use the toilet. Alternatively, it might be possible to help the individual find a method of communicating this desire. In patients who are unaware of the need to void, then a programme to establish a routine for toileting based on the patient's bladder chart can be highly successful in most cases.

A neurogenic bladder due to damage or impairment

between the cerebral cortex micturating control centre and the bladder can arise for a variety of reasons – dementia, cerebrovascular accident, multiple sclerosis, cerebral palsy, tumour, Parkinson's disease, spinal cord injury, spina bifida, diabetic neuropathy. The type of incontinence will vary according to the site and extent of the damage (see Chapter 2), and can be established by careful history and assessment. Some patients have difficulty in emptying their bladder completely and thus risk developing a persistent urinary tract infection. Residual urine can also result in overflow incontinence.

A good fluid intake of 2–3 litres/day is especially important in patients who are paralysed, or those who may develop a small bladder syndrome. Patients with paralysis may not experience the normal sensation and conscious desire to void; however they can usually trigger a reflex action at will, providing the sacral nerves are intact. Methods used include tapping or kneading the abdominal wall between the symphysis pubis and umbilicus to initiate and often sustain voiding if the reflex is poor. Pulling the pubic hair or stroking the inside of the thighs can work for some people. Pressure on the perineum or anal stimulation has also been used successfully by some patients. In practice it is best to discuss the various methods of stimulation with individual patients and for them to experiment, if they wish, to find one that is acceptable and works for them. Sometimes a patient may try either a Valsalva or Credé technique; the former involves increasing the abdominal pressure by taking a deep breath then closing the glottis and forcefully exhaling and straining. However, the mechanics of this technique are not to be recommended for use in the long term and never in patients suspected of sphincter spasm or resistance, as damage to the musculature of the pelvic floor and surrounding tissue can occur. The Credé technique involves manual expression of the bladder, by clenching the fist and applying direct pressure to the abdominal wall.

References

Azrin N. H., Fox R. M. (1974). *Toilet Training in Less Than a Day.* London: Pan.

Bakwin H. (1983). The genetics of bedwetting. In *Bladder Control and Enuresis*. (Kolvin I., MacKeith R. C., Meadow S. R., eds). London: Spastics International Medical Publications Heinemann.

Blackwell B., Currah J. (1973). The psychopharmacology of nocturnal enuresis. In *Bladder Control and Enuresis*. (Kolvin I., MacKeith R. C., Meadow S. R., eds). London: Spastics International Medical Publications, Heinemann.

Broomfield J. W., Douglas J. W. B. (1956). Bedwetting prevalence among children aged 4–7 years. *Lancet*, i, 850–2.

Castleden C. M., Duffin H. M., Asher M. J. et al, (1986). Factors influencing outcome in elderly patients with urinary incontinence and detrusor instability. *Age and Ageing*, 14, 303–7.

Clay E. C. (1978). Incontinence of urine. *Nursing Mirror*, 146 (14), 36–8; 146 (11), 23–4.

Henry M. (1983). Faecal incontinence. *Nursing Times*, August 17, 61–2.

King M. (1980). Treatment of incontinence. *Nursing Times*, 76, 1006–10.

Kolvin I., MacKeith R. C., Medows S. R. (eds) (1973). Bladder control and enuresis. London: Heinemann Medical Books.

Landman G. B., Rappaport L. (1985). Paediatric management of severe treatment resistant encopresis. *Development and Behavioural Paediatrics*, 6, 6.

Lask B. (1977). Emotional and behavioural problems in childhood. *Midwife, Health Visitor and Community Nurse*, 13, 363–5.

Meadow R. (1980). Help for bedwetting. Edinburgh: Churchill Livingstone.

Morgan R. T. T. (1978). Relapse and therapeutic response in the conditioning treatment of enuresis. A review of recent findings on intermittent reinforcement overlearning stimulus intensity. *Behavioural Research and Therapy*, 16, 273–9.

Norton C. (1986). *Nursing for Continence* Beaconsfield: Beaconsfield Publishers.

Robbins B. (1985). The psychology of incontinence. *Journal of District Nursing*, 16, 36–7.

Rutter M., Yule W., Graham P. (1973). Enuresis and behavioural deviance: some epidemiological considerations. In *Bladder Control and Enuresis*. (Kolvin I., MacKeith R. C., Meadow S. R., eds). London: Spastics Society International Medical Publications, Heinemann.

Shaffer D. (1976). Nocturnal enuresis. *Nursing Times*, 72, 616–18.

Simmonds J. F. (1977). *Clinical Paediatrics*, 16, 79–82.

Sillitoe R., Reed S. (1986). Enuresis – dry at night. *Community Outlook*, March 20.

Sole G. H., James G. (1984). The presentation and management of elderly patients with chronic retention. *Journal of Clinical Experimental Gerontology*, 3, 191–9.
Stone H. (1983). *Adult Bedwetters and their Problems: A Road to Homelessness*. Canterbury: Cyrenians.
Tarrier N., Larner S. (1983). The effects of manipulation of social reinforcement on toilet requests on a geriatric ward. *Age and Ageing*, 12, 234–9.
Thomas T. M., Plymat K. R., Blannin J. et al (1980). The prevalence of urinary incontinence. *British Medical Journal*, 281, 1243–5.
Tierney A. J. (1973). Toilet training. *Nursing Times*, 69, 1740–5.
Timmreck T. G. (1983). Behavioural therapy for night bedwetting in children with parents as therapists. *Journal of Psychosocial Nursing*.
Tobin G. W., Brocklehurst J. C. (1986a). Faecal incontinence in residential homes for the elderly: prevalence, aetiology and management. *Age and Ageing*, 15, 41–6.
Tobin G. W., Brocklehurst J. G. (1986b). The management of urinary incontinence in local authority residential homes for elderly. *Age and Ageing*, 15, 292–8.
Turner R. K., Young G. C., Rochman S. (1980). Treatment of nocturnal enuresis by conditioning techniques. *Behaviour Research and Therapy*, 8, 367–81.
Wishart M. C., Bidder R. T. (1981). Enuresis: present trends in treatment. *Health Visitor*, 54, 532–3.

Bibliography

Bowley A. H., Gardner L. (1980). *The Handicapped Child*. London: Churchill Livingstone.
Essen J., Packham C. (1976). Nocturnal enuresis in childhood development. *Medical and Child Neurology*, 18, 577–89.
Millard D. M. (1984). *Daily Living with a Handicapped Child*. Kent: Croom Helm.
Morgan R. T. T. (1981). *Childhood Incontinence*. London: Heinemann Medical Books.
Russell P. (1984). *The Wheelchair Child* 2nd edn. London: Human Horizon Series, Souvenir Press.

Index

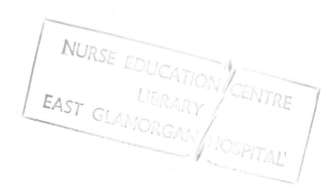